NUTRITION AND DIET RESEARCH PROGRESS

DOES VITAMIN C ACT AS AN ANTIOXIDANT OR PROOXIDANT?

MÜFIDE AYDOGAN

AND

ASLI KORKMAZ

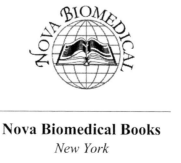

Nova Biomedical Books

New York

Library of Congress Cataloging-in-Publication Data
Aydogan, M|fide.
  Does vitamin C act as an antioxidant or prooxidant? / M|fide Aydogan, Asli Korkmaz.
     p. ; cm.
  Includes bibliographical references and index.
  ISBN 978-1-61761-096-7 (softcover)
  1. Vitamin C--Physiological effect. 2. Antioxidants. 3. Oxidizing agents. I. Korkmaz, Asli. II. Title.
  [DNLM: 1. Ascorbic Acid--pharmacology. 2. Antioxidants--pharmacology. QU 210]
  QP772.A8A93 2010
  612.3'99--dc22   2010027277

Published by Nova Science Publishers, Inc. † New York

90 0900828 0

7 DAY | CT AS AN
)OXIDANT?

NUTRITION AND DIET RESEARCH PROGRESS

Additional books in this series can be found on Nova's website under the Series tab.

Additional E-books in this series can be found on Nova's website under the E-book tab

Contents

Preface

Vitamin C is known to be an effective antioxidant in biological fluids and cells, and generally believed to be beneficial components from vegetables and fruits. Vitamin C is an important dietary antioxidant which significantly decreases the adverse effects of reactive oxygen species (ROS) formed in the cell. Paradoxically, vitamin C has also been shown to oxidize the cellular components under certain *in vitro* experimental conditions and induce cell death in a number of different cell lines. However, the mechanism of the oxidizing feature of vitamin C is not well understood. It has been reported that vitamin C loses its effectiveness as antioxidant at high concentrations or at partial oxygen pressures. Some data concluded that vitamin C acts as an prooxidant rather than antioxidant. It was reported that vitamin C administrated as a dietary supplement to healthy humans exhibits a prooxidant, as well as an antioxidant, effect *in vivo*. *In vitro* studies demonstrated that vitamin C is reactive with metal ions and produces the ascorbate radicals which causes oxidative damage to biomolecules. The mixtures of ascorbate-iron administration have been shown to stimulate free radical damage to DNA, lipids and proteins *in vitro*. It has been suggested of importance by observational epidemiologic that antioxidant vitamins, containing vitamin C, at an effective doses inhibit heart disease and cancer. Ascorbate has been reported to induce apoptotic cell death, characterized by cell shrinkage, nuclear fragmentation and internucleosomal DNA cleavage, in human myelogenous leukemic cell lines by acting anticancerogenic and prooxidative manner. In addition, some *in vivo* studies showed that vitamin C co-administration along with environmental chemicals, which cause oxidative damage in tissues, aggravates this oxidative damage in the tissues of rats. After started an oxidative damage, vitamin C administration could promote the damage and be prooxidant depending on the environment and conditions in which the molecule is active. The purpose of the present manuscript is to exhibit the antioxidant and especially prooxidant effects of vitamin C.

Chapter I

Introduction
Historical Overview

The earlier sailors developed a weird disease called scurvy when they were on sea. The disease scurvy which is now known to be the result of vitamin C (L-Ascorbic acid) deficiency was described by the ancient Greeks, Egyptians and Romans and has long been associated with capturing armies, navies and explorers. In 1536 the French explorer Jacques Cartier described that nature of this disease. By the late 1700s' the British navy was aware that scurvy could be cured by eating fresh citrus fruits. The definition of scurvy could have been selected from descriptions published several years ago. For example, McCord [1] defined scurvy in his publication as a "a condition due to deficiency of vitamin C in the diet and marked by weakness, anemia, spongy gums, offensive breath, bleeding and bruising easily, hair and tooth loss, joint pain and swelling, livid spots on the skin, general debility, and a pale bloated countenance, brawny indurations of the muscles of the legs". Such symptoms appear to be related to the weakening of blood vessels, connective tissue, and bone, which all contain collagen. Vitamin C was first isolated from natural sources by Szent-Gyorgyi, [2] who was awarded the Nobel Prize for the discovery of vitamin C. A few months later Reichstein et al. [3] determined the precise structure of vitamin C. At that time, however, little molecular explanation for the vitamin C was available. Until today, many studies have been made about the structure, bioavailability, effects etc. of vitamin C.

Chemistry of Ascorbic Acid

Structurally, vitamin C or ascorbic acid is one of the simplest vitamins. It was first isolated form cabbage, orange and adrenal glands as an acidic carbohydrate [2]. Ascorbate has two ionizable –OH groups. Since it is a mono-anion is the favored from at physiological pH [4, 5].The physical properties of vitamin C are seen Table 1.

Ascorbate is an excellent reducing agent. It readily undergoes two consecutive, yet reversible, one-electron oxidation processes to generate the ascorbyl radical (A$^{\bullet -}$) as an intermediate and dehydroascorbic acid (DHA) (Figure1). Ascorbyl radical is a relatively unreactive free radical because its reduction potential is considerably low compared to other radicals such as α-tocopherol radical, the gluthatione radical and all reactive oxygen and nitrogen species that are thought to be involved in human disease [6]. These properties make ascorbate a superior biological donor antioxidant.

Table 1. Physical properties of vitamin C

Properties	Explanations
Chemical Formula	$C_6H_8O_6$
Molecular weight	176.13
Appererance	White, crystalline solid, acidic taste, inodorous
m.p. (°C)	190- 192
Dencity (g/ml)	1.65
pH	3 (50 mg/ml)
PK$_{a1}$	4.25
Pk$_{a2}$	11.8
Redox potential	First stage: $E_1O+ 0.166V$
Water solubility g/ml	0.33
Fats and oils solubility	insoluble

As can be seen in Table 2, ascorbate is thermodinamically at the bottom of pecking order of oxidizing free radicals. That is, all oxidizing free radicals with greater reduction potentials, which includes HO$^{\bullet}$, RO$^{\bullet}$, LOO$^{\bullet}$, GS$^{\bullet}$, urate, and even the tocopheroxyl radical (TO$^{\bullet}$), can be repaired by ascorbate. From Table 2, it can be seen that the kinetics of these electron (hydrogen atom) transfer reactions are rapid. Thus, both thermodynamically and kinetically, ascorbate can be considered to be an excellent antioxidant.

Ascorbate is readily oxidized. However, the rate of this oxidation is dependent upon pH and presence of catalytic metals. The diacid is very slow to oxidize. Consequently, at low pH (<2 or 3), ascorbic acid solutions are quite stable, assuming catalytic transition metal ions are not introduced into the solutions. However, as the pH is raised above pK_1, AH^- becomes dominant and the stability of the ascorbate solution decreases. The loss of the stability is usually the result of the adventitious catalytic metals in buffer and salts that are typically employed in studies at near neutral pH. In carefully demetalled solutions, as the pH is varied, the rate of oxidation increases (Figure 2).

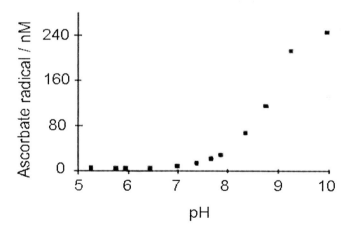

Ascorbic Acid (AA)   Ascorbate (AH⁻)   Ascorbyl Radical (A˙⁻)   Dehydroascorbic Acid (DHA)

Figure 1. Redox metabolism of vitamin C. The electron oxidation of ascorbate generates ascorbate radical which on further oxidation forms dehydroascorbic acid. Dehydroascorbic acid is an unstable molecule and can be decomposed or reduced back to ascorbate (Adapted from reference 6) .

Figure 2. Background Asc˙ vs. pH: Each solution was made with 50 mM demetalled phosphate buffer that contained 50 μM desferoxamine mesylate, for at least 12 h. To these solutions 500 μM ascorbate was added and the EPR spectra were collected. The points represent the Asc˙ concentration observed in the second of three EPR scans, where the values had a Standard deviation of less than 1 nanomolar [8].

Table 2. One-Electron Reduction Potentials at pH 7.0 for Selected Radical Couples (Adapted from reference 7)

	Couple	Standard Reduction Potential (mv)
Highly	$HO^{\bullet}$, H^{+}/H_2O	2310
Oxidizing	$RO^{\bullet}$, H^{+}/ROH (aliphatic alkoxyl)	1600
	$HO_2^{\bullet}$, H^{+}/H_2O_2	1060
	$O_2^{\bullet}$, $2H^{+}/H_2O_2$	940
	$RS^{\bullet}$, RS (cysteine)	920
	$HU^{\bullet}$, H^{+}/UH_2 (urate)	590
	$\alpha T^{\bullet}$, $H^{+}/\alpha TH$ (α-tocopherol)	500
	Trolox C ($TO^{\bullet}$,H^{+}/TOH)	480
	H_2O_2 H^{+}/H_2O, $HO^{\bullet}$	320
	Ascorbate$^{\bullet}$, $H^{+}/$ Ascorbate^{-}	282
	Ferricytochrome c/ferrocytochrome c	260
	Ubisemiquinone, Hflubiquinol	200
	Fe^{3+}- EDTA/Fe^{2+}- EDTA	120
	Fe^{3+}citrate/Fe^{2+}citrate	~100
	Fe^{3+}-ADP/Fe^{2+}-AD	~100
	Ubiquinone, $H^{+}/$ubisemiquinone	-36
	Dehydroascorbate/ascorbate$^{\bullet}$	**-174**
	Fe^{3+} - ferritin/ferritin + Fe^{2+}	-190
	$O_2/O_2^{\bullet}$	-330
	Fe^{3+} - transferrin/Fe2+-transferrin	-400 (pH 7.3)
	Paraquat/paraquat$^{\bullet}$	-448
	O_2/H^{+}, $HO_2^{\bullet}$	-460
Highly	$CO_2/CO_2^{\bullet}$	-1800
Reducing	H_2O/e_{aq}	-2840

Ascorbate is now known that because it is at the bottom of pecking order for oxidizing free radicals, it will serve as a donor andioxidant to repair each of the oxidizing radicals above it. The tocopheroxyl radical has a reduction potential of around +500 mV, thus it will be repaired by ascorbate with follows reaction:

$$TO^{\bullet} + AH^{-} \rightarrow TOH + A^{\bullet -} \ (k= 2 \times 10^{5} \ M^{-1}s^{-1})$$

Biosynthesis of Vitamin C

Biosynthesis of vitamin C was a relatively late event in evolution. Since vitamin C is not present in E. coli or other bacteria. Most of plants and animals synthesize Vitamin C from glucose (Figure 3). A majority of animals produce relatively high levels of vitamin C. The location of vitamin C biosynthesis is interesting issue. In primitive fishes, amphibians and reptiles vitamin C synthesis takes place in kidneys, whereas the liver is the site of synthesis in mammals [9]. A more complex situation is observed in birds, where all two conditions have been observed (kidney, liver) [10]. In plants, virtually all cells synthesize vitamin C, but the synthesis is much higher in meristematic cells [11].

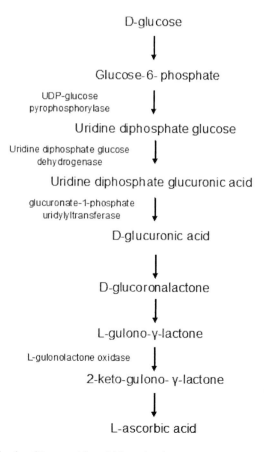

Figure 3. Biosynthesis of L-ascorbic acid in animals.

Guinea pigs, fruit bats, humans and other primates have lost the ability to synthesize vitamin C as a result of a mutation in the gene coding for L-gulonolactone oxidase, an enzyme required for the biosynthesis of vitamin C via the glucuronic acid pathway [12]. The gene encoding GuLO was found to be present in the human genome, but not expressed due to the accumulation of a number of mutations [13]. Even in vertebrates capable of synthesizing vitamin C, biosynthesis only takes place in a few cell types. Hence, in humans vitamin C has to be supplemented through food and or as tablets. Consequently, when humans do not ingest vitamin C in their diets, a deficiency state occurs with a wide spectrum of clinical manifestations. Thus, humans must ingest vitamin C to survive.

Catabolism of Vitamin C

Mammalian cells take vitamin C from tissue fluids against concentration gradient coupled to uptake of sodium. Absorption of vitamin C occurs primarily in the distal small intestine via active transport through an vitamin C transporter termed the sodium-dependent vitamin C transporter-type 1. This transporter is also present in the renal proximal tubules, where it serves to reabsorb filtered vitamin C [14]. It has been suggested that the transfer of the vitamin C biosynthetic machinery in animals from the kidney of cold blooded reptiles to the much larger and more active liver of mammals reflected the increased need for vitamin C due to increasing atmospheric oxygen [15].

Vitamin C being a water soluble compound is easily absorbed but it is not stored in the body. The average adult has a body pool of 1.2–2.0 g of vitamin C. The first degradation product of vitamin C is semidehydroascorbic acid or ascorbyl radical. Ascorbyl radical, with its unpaired electron, is not a long lived compound. Upon loss of a second electron, the compound formed is dehydroascorbic acid. Dehydroascorbic acid stability depends on factors such as temperature and pH, but is often only minutes [16]. Vitamin C/dehydroascorbic acid ratios seem to be kept very high in body fluids and tissues during health, i.e. almost no dehydroascorbic acid. This ratio has been reported to fall in some diseases, including diabetes and rheumatoid arthritis [17]. Once formed, ascorbyl radical $(A^{\bullet-})$ and dehydroascorbic acid can be reduced back to vitamin C by at least three separate enzyme pathways as well as by reducing compounds in biological systems such as reduced glutathione.

Ascorbate can be recycled by chemical and enzymatic mechanism. A$^{\bullet-}$ can be converted back to vitamin C by an NADH-dependent reductase or by dismutation of two-molecules of the radical into one molecule of vitamin C and one molecule of DHA. DHA can be reduced back to ascorbate either directly by glutathione or enzymatically by a glutathione-dependent DHA reductase, glutaredoxin, or the NADPH-dependent thioredoxin reductase (Figure 4) [6].

If dehydroascorbic acid is not reduced back to vitamin C, it is hydrolyzed to 2,3 diketogulonic acid which is formed by irreversible rupture of the lactone ring structure that is a part of vitamin C, ascorbyl radical, and dehydroascorbic acid. 2,3-diketogulonic acid is further metabolized into xylose, xylonate, lyxonate and oxalate [18]. The main route of elimination of vitamin C and its metabolites is through urine. It is excreted unchanged when high doses of vitamin C are consumed. The formation of oxalate has clinical significance because there is some concern that high vitamin C intake could increase the risk of oxalate kidney stones [19].

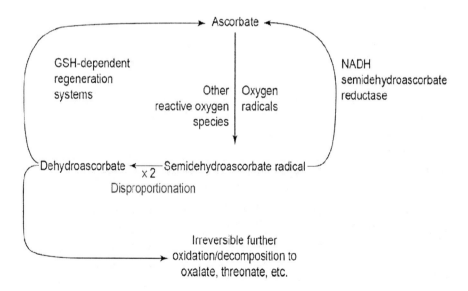

Figure 4. Oxidation, regeneration and decomposition of ascorbate. Two semidehydroascorbate radicals can undergo dismutation to produce ascorbate and dehydroascorbate. GSH, reduced glutathione [20].

Recommended Dietary Allowance (RDA) of Vitamin C

In 1974, Recommended Dietary Allowance (RDA) of vitamin C has been set at 45 mg/day for adults, 35 mg/day for infants, 60 mg/day for pregnant women, and 80 mg/day for lactating mothers by the Food and Nutrition Board of the National Academy of Science-U.S.National Research Council [21]. The RDA is determined by the rate of turnover and rate of depletion of an initial body pool of 1500 mg vitamin C and an assumed absorption of <85% of the vitamin at usual intakes. The RDA continues to be based primarily on the prevention of deficiency disease, rather than the prevention of chronic disease and the promotion of optimum health. The RDA for vitamin C was revised in 2000 upward from the previous recommendation of 60 mg daily for healthy, non smoking adults [22]. However, the preventative functions of vitamin C in cardiovascular disease, certain cancers etc, provide compelling arguments for an increase in dietary intakes and RDAs [23]. Bendich and Langseth [24] found that populations consuming more than 60 mg/day of vitamin C from diet or supplements had a reduced risk of cancers, cardiovascular disease, and cataracts. Similarly, it has been suggested that a dietary intake of 100 mg/day of vitamin C is associated with reduced incidence of mortality from heart diseases, stroke and cancer [25].

Plant Food Sources of Vitamin C

Vitamin C is widely distributed in fresh fruits and vegetables. Since it is not difficult to obtain an adequate supply in the daily diet. As shown in Table 3, relatively high amount of vitamin C are found in rosehip, strawberries, citrus fruits, and various vegetables, although the availability of vitamin C within these food sources will be influenced by numerous factors [26-28].

Table 3. Vitamin C content in selected fruit and vegetables (changed from Ref. 23-25)

Source	mg/ 100 g
Apple	2-30
Apricot	7-10
Avacado	15-20
Banana	8-30
Broccoli	110
Brussels sprout	90-120
Cabbage	30-45
Cauliflower	50-78
Carrot	6
Cherry	5-15
Redcurrant	40
Blackcurrant	150-200
Egg plant	15-20
Gooseberry	40
Grapefruit	40-70
Horseradish	120
Kiwi	60
Lemon	40-50
Lime	25
Loganberry	30
Melon	10-35
Orange	50
Onion	10-15
Parsley	200-300
Peach	10-30
Pear	4
Pepper	150-200
Plum	3
Pineapple	10- 25
Potato	10-30
Raspberry	25
Rosehip	1000
Spinach	35-40
Strawberry	40-70
Tangerine	30
Tomato	10-20

Chapter II

Biological Functions of Vitamin C in Animals

One of the more clearly defined functions of vitamin C in both plant and animal metabolism is to modulate a number of important enzymatic reactions. Since vitamin C acts as an electron donor for different enzymes [29]. Typically, these enzymes are mono- or dioxygenases, which contain iron or copper at the active site and which require vitamin C for maximal activity. [30,31]. Vitamin C accelerates hydroxylation reactions by maintaining the active center of metal ions in a reduced state for optimal activity of enzymes hydroxylase and oxygenase [32].These enzymes are necessary for synthesis of collogen, carnitine, norepinephrine.

Procollagen-proline dioxygenase (proline hydroxylase) and procollagen-lysine 5-dioxygenase (lysine hydroxylase), two enzymes involved in procollagen biosynthesis, require vitamin C for maximal activity [33]. The hydroxylation reactions add hydroxyl groups to the amino acids proline or lysine in the collagen molecule, thereby greatly increasing stability of the collagen molecule triple helix structure. Collagen represents about one third of the total body protein. It constitutes the principal protein of connective tissue framework of entire body including skin, bones, teeth, cartilage, tendons, blood vessels, heart valves, inter vertebral discs, cornea and eye lens.

Two dioxygenases (gamma Butyrobetaine 2-oxoglutarate 4-dioxygenase, Trimethyllysine 2-oxoglutarate dioxygenase) involved in the biosynthesis of carnitine also require vitamin C as a cofactor for maximal activity [34]. Carnitine is essential for the transport of fatty acids into mitochondria where it can be used for energy production. In addition, vitamin C is used as a cofactor for catecholamine biosynthesis, in particular the biosynthesis of norepinephrine from dopamine catalyzed by dopamine b-monooxygenase [35].

Vitamin C is also necessary for the transformation of cholesterol to bile acids as it modulates the microsomal 7 α-hydroxylation, the rate limiting reaction of cholesterol catabolism in liver. Further, vitamin C catalyzes other enzymatic reactions involving amidation necessary for maximal activity of hormones oxytocin, vasopressin, cholecystokinin and alpha-melanotripin [36].

Iron and copper are essential in the human body for the synthesis of huge range of enzymes and other proteins involved in respiration, oxygen transport, nitric oxide formation and other redox reactions. Vitamin C is known to enhance the availability and absorption of iron from the small intestine by keeping iron reduced. This effect is seen at vitamin C doses of 20–60 mg, an amount easily found in one meal of healthy diets [37].On the other hand reduction of metal ions such as iron or copper by vitamin C *in vitro* can result in the formation of highly reactive hydroxyl radicals via reaction of the reduced metal ions with hydrogen peroxide, a process known as Fenton chemistry [38].

Generation of reactive oxygen species (ROS) such as superoxide radical (O_2^-), hydrogen peroxide (H_2O_2), and hydroxyl radical (OH^-) is a normal process in aerobic organisms, but at the same time an internal threat to cellular homeostasis can arise from these reactive oxygen intermediates and the by-products generated from oxygen metabolism [39]. ROS cause significant oxidative damage by attacking biomolecules such as membrane lipids, DNA, and proteins in cells [40]. Oxidative damage to these biomolecules has been implicated in many chronic diseases, such as cardiovascular disease, cancer, atherosclerosis and cataract [41]. Antioxidants neutralize ROS by donating one of their own electrons, ending the electron-"stealing" reaction. They act as scavengers, helping to prevent cell and tissue damage that could lead to cellular damage and disease. Aerobic organisms have developed a range of efficient mechanisms to detoxify ROS by enzymatic (catalase CAT, superoxide dismutase SOD, and glutathione peroxidase GPx) means. SOD is the first antioxidant enzyme to deal with ROS by accelerating the dismutation of O_2^- to H_2O_2. CAT is a peroxiosomal heam protein that catalyses the removal of H_2O_2 formed during the reaction catalysed by SOD. GPx catalyses the reduction of H_2O_2 to water and O_2^- at the expence of reduced glutathione (GSH). Low-molecular-weight antioxidants such as GSH vitamin C,vitamin E, as well as carotenoids and phenolics are able to nonenzymically interact directly with ROS [42,43]. The most striking chemical property of vitamin C is it is ability to act as a radical (i.e. ROS) scavenger. Thus, as an electron donor, vitamin C is a powerful water-soluble antioxidant in humans.

Although all molecules are susceptible to ROS injury, lipids are targeted most frequently. Several studies have demonstrated that ROS can produce cellular injury by attacking membranes through peroxidation of polyunsaturated fatty acids that can alter both membrane structure and function of mitochondrial, lysosomal, and cell membrane via lipid peroxidation [44,45]. Malondialdehyde (MDA) is an end product of lipid peroxidation and widely accepted as a marker of ROS-mediated lipid peroxidation in the cell [46].Proteins also undergo oxidation by several mechanisms [47,48]. A peptide chain can be cleaved by oxidants, or specific amino acids can be oxidized. Protein oxidation most commonly is measured by detection of modified groups (carbonyl groups) or the oxidized amino acids themselves. ROS can lead to DNA damage by direct chemical attack on DNA, and also by indirect mechanism. Indirect mechanisms leading to DNA damage include protein oxidation, which could alter repair enzymes and DNA polymerases. An increasingly popular marker of *in vivo* oxidative damage to DNA is 8-oxoguanine (8-oxoG) [49].

Chapter III

Antioxidant Effect of Vitamin C on Diseases

During the past two decade, it has become apparent that free radical damage may contribute to cellular dysfunction and disease and oxidative damage has been implicated in a number of pathological processes, including carcinogenesis, cardiovascular disease, cataracts, neurodegenerative diseases and diabetes mellitus arthritis, adult respiratory-distress syndrome, emphysema, retinopathy of prematurity, aging, atherosclerosis, muscular dystrophy, and ischemia-reperfusion tissue injury [20,50].When reactive oxygen species (ROS) and reactive nitrogen species (RNS) are generated in living systems, a wide variety of antioxidants comes into play [42].

In general, these natural antioxidants, like vitamin C and E, carotenoids, and flavonoids, are considered to be beneficial components from fruit and vegetables. The antioxidative properties of these compounds are often claimed to be responsible for the protective effects of these food components against cardiovascular disease, certain forms of cancer and/or photosensitivity diseases [51-56]. Besides, a large body of epidemiological studies has shown that populations with a high intake of antioxidants, including ascorbic acid, vitamin E and flavonoids have a lower rate of cardiovascular diseases than populations with low intake [57]. Fruits and vegetable consumption decreases the amount of free-radical damage to DNA in the human body (a risk factor of cancer development), but supplements of ascorbate, vitamin E, or β-carotene do not decrease DNA damage in most studies [58-62].

Atherosclerosis and Cardiovascular Disease

Many scientists report low-density lipoprotein (LDL) oxidation as the main reason for atherosclerosis [63] In spite of several mechanisms that had been proposed to explain the pathogenesis of atherosclerosis, most of the attention has focused on the role of ROS. LDL, the major carrier of cholesterol and lipids in the blood, infiltrates the intima of arterial sites, where it is oxidized over time by oxidants generated by local vascular cells [64]. Adhesion of leukocytes to the endothelium is an important step in initiating atherosclerosis. The oxidized LDL further inhibits the egress of macrophages from the artery wall, where the cells recognize and readily take up the oxidized LDL through a process mediated by scavenger receptors. Vitamin C protects against oxidation of isolated LDL by different types of oxidative stress, including metal ion dependent and independent processes [65]. For example, LDL is isolated from plasma and then subjected to oxidation conditions, in the presence of a transition metal (copper or iron). Delay in oxidation by vitamin C is measured as lag time and change in rate of lipid peroxidation [66]. In addition, *in vitro* studies have shown that physiological concentrations of vitamin C strongly inhibit LDL oxidation by vascular endothelial cells [67]. Furthermore, derivatives of vitamin C showed protective effect on lipid-peroxide induced endothelial injury [63]. *In vivo* studies have indicated that vitamin C inhibits leukocyte-endothelial cell interactions induced by cigarette smoke [68,69] or oxidized LDL [70]. Dietary antioxidants can decrease atherosclerosis in LDL receptor deficient mice, cholesterol fed rabbits and cholesterol fed primates [71-73]. For example, animals can be fed high cholesterol diets with induction of atherosclerosis, which was decreased by antioxidants including vitamins C and E [74,75]. Overall, both *in vitro* and *in vivo* experiments showed that vitamin C protects isolated LDL and plasma lipid peroxidation induced by various radical or ROS. In studies with human plasma lipids it was shown that vitamin C was far more effective in inhibiting lipid peroxidation initiated by a peroxyl radical initiator than other plasma components, such as protein thiols, urate, bilirubin, and a-tocopherol. Thus, by efficiently trapping peroxyl radicals in the aqueous phase before they can initiate lipid peroxidation, vitamin C can protect biomembranes against peroxidative damage [76]. Vitamin C can also act to protect membranes against peroxidation by enhancing the activity of tocopherol, the chain-breaking antioxidant. With *in vitro* studies it was shown that vitamin C reduces the tocopheroxyl radical and thereby restores the radical-scavenging activity of tocopherol [77,78]. In short, atherosclerosis is a disease of initial inflammation and subsequent oxidative damage. Since vitamin C has the potential to counteract both of these processes, it represents a practical solution for the early prevention of the disease.

High blood pressure, hypertension, is a well-established risk factor for cardiovascular disease (CVD). It presumably facilities injury to the vascular endothelium by increasing stress caused by following blood [79]. The pathogenesis of hypertension can involve genetic factors and exposing to toxins including cigarette smoke. Further, some evidence suggests that increased vascular oxidative stress contributes to the pathophysiology of endothelial dysfunction and hypertension [80,81]. Low plasma vitamin C concentrations have been associated with hypertension and impaired endothelial function. Since vitamin C may increase endothelial nitric oxide (NO) by protecting it from oxidation [82]. NO which produced by endothelial nitric oxide sythase (eNOS) is an important vasodilator molecule regulating vascular tonus in human. So, vitamin C and the other antioxidant vitamin, vitamin E, appear to have beneficial effects on vascular endothelial function in healthy subjects and in patients with cardiovascular disease. However, a recent analysis on the role of vitamin C and antioxidant vitamins showed no evidence of significant benefit in prevention of CHD [83].

Cancer

Basic research has shown that radical damage (oxidation) to cellular components (i.e. DNA) likely plays an important role in carcinogenesis. DNA oxidation can lead to deleterious mutations which are the initiating events in neoplasms [84,85]. Most oxidative lesions are efficiently repaired by specific DNA glycosylases, but repair is not completely efficient and the number of lesions accumulates with age. When the cells divide, the lesions become fixated and mutations and cancer may result [86]. Because of this, DNA oxidation is thought to increase the incidence of cancers. A large number of epidemiologic studies have shown that dietary intake of antioxidant vitamins, mainly from fruit and vegetables, protects against different types of cancer [87,88]. In 1970's it was believed that vitamin C fights cancer by promoting collagen synthesis and thus prevents tumors from invading the surrounding tissues [89]. However, researchers currently believe that vitamin C prevents cancer by neutralizing ROS before they can damage DNA and initiate tumor growth and or may act as a pro-oxidant helping body's own free radicals to destroy tumors in their early stages [90,91]. In addition, vitamin C may reduce carcinogenesis through stimulation of the immune system. Free radicals and ROS secreted by cytotoxic T lymphocytes, macrophages, and natural killer cells can lyse tumor cells. Vitamin C can protect host cells against harmful oxidants released into the extracellular medium [92].

Numerous reports are available in literature on cytotoxic and anti-carcinogenic effect of vitamin C *in vitro* and *in vivo* systems. However, the molecular mechanisms underlying the anti-carcinogenic potential of vitamin C are not completely elucidated. Some of these studies have been located in this chapter. One of the most consistent epidemiological findings on vitamin C has been an association with high intake of vitamin C rich foods and reduced risk of stomach cancer. Normally, the concentration of vitamin C in gastric juice is approximately three times higher than that of plasma. Yet, vitamin C content is low in the gastric juice of patients with hypochlorhydria, atrophic gastritis and Helicobacter pylori infection, conditions associated with gastric cancer. Further, elimination of the bacteria increases gastric vitamin C secretion [93]. Gastric juice ascorbate may be an important scavenger of such species as peroxynitrite (ONOO-) and hypochlorous acid (HOCl), and its decreases the formation of carcinogenic N-nitroso compounds by reaction of RNS [94]. Similarly Helser et al. [95] shown that formation of nitrosamines in the gastrointestinal tract can be decreased by administration of vitamin C.

Orally administration of vitamin C significantly inhibited human mammary tumor growth in mice [96]. Further, vitamin C and its derivatives were shown to be cytotoxic and inhibited the growth of a number of malignant and non-malignant cell lines *in vitro* and *in vivo* [97]. Also, vitamin C has been reported to be cytotoxic to some human tumor cells including, neuorblastoma [98], osteosarcoma and retinoblastoma [99]. The incidence of kidney tumors decreased by vitamin C in hamsters due to decrease in the formation of genotoxic metabolites [100].

Ischemia/Reperfusion Injury

Ischemia due to arterial occlusion or organ transplantation is a common cause of renal cell death and organ failure and, in the case of transplantation, of delayed graft function or graft rejection. Reperfusion aggravates the damage [101]. The mechanisms proposed to explain warm I/R injury include anoxia, release of ROS during reperfusion, neutrophil accumulation, and subsequent release of additional ROS and lytic enzymes [102]. Many studies have shown that antioxidants act as protective against I/R induced cell damage. In our previous study, we tried to determine the possible protective effect of vitamin C, as an antioxidant, against I/R-induced acute renal failure in the kidney of rats [103]. The result of the functional parameters, oxidative stress markers, and histological changes suggest that vitamin C play a role in a decrease in I/R-induced injury and assist in the recovery of the renal function after renal I/R. Pre-treatment of kidney transplant recipients with a vitamin C solution led to better early graft function [104]. Also vitamin C has been reported to reduce I/R induced oxidative stress in the cardiac and liver tissues of rats [105,106]. Vitamin C has an especially large range of doses, from 30 mg/kg to 1,000 mg/kg on I/R studies. But the hepatoprotective effects against I/R induced injury were only shown in the rats treated with low dose (30–100 mg/kg) [103]. Further, vitamin C was shown to cross the blood brain barrier by means of facilitative transport and was suggested to offer neuroprotection against cerebral ischemia by augmenting antioxidant levels of brain [107].

Wound Healing

Healing of a wound is a complex and protracted process of tissue repair and remodeling in response to injury. All phases of wound healing (inflamation, proliferation and maturation) are either directly or indirectly controlled by several enzymes. Vitamin C is critical in wound healing, acting as a cofactor for collagen stabilizing enzymes, including lysyl and prolyl hydroxylase [108]. Also vitamin C differentially regulates elastin biosynthsis in vascular smooth muscle cells. Adequate supplies of vitamin C are necessary for normal healing process especially for post-operative patients. If vitamin C deficiency occurs, fibroblasts cannot produce stable collagen, providing a weak framework for repair, thus impairing wound healing [109]. It has been suggest that vitamin C intake accelerates the synthesis of collogen at the site of wound or burn trauma. Hellman and Burn [110] recommended that administration of 1 g/day of vitamin C accelerates the wound healing. Generally, vitamin C levels are low in older patients, which may contribute to slower and more difficult wound healing. It was reported that vitamin C counteracted a reduced proliferative capacity of elderly dermal fibroblasts *in vivo* [109].

Cataract

Cataract is thought to result, at least in part from oxidative damages to lens proteins which, leading cause of blindness in the world. UV light and ionizing radiation often induce cataract, perhaps by increased formation of OH^- and other ROS [111]. Vitamin C is present at high concentration in the lens, cornea, retinal pigment epithelium and aqueous humor of human, monkey and other animals [112]. The lens epithelium actively transports sodium ions (Na^+) ions out of the lens, and potassium ions (K^+) into it, using and ion-transporting ATPase. Lens epithelial cells are readily damaged by ROS, showing DNA strand breakage and abnormalities of ion transport, i.e. damage to the Na^+-K^+ ATPase. Vitamin C protects the lens ion transporting ATPase against damage by ROS generating system *in vitro* [113]. Several epidemiologic studies have investigated the association of vitamin C intake with the incidence of cataract. For example Hankinson et al. [114] showed that vitamin C (260mg/day) has a protective effect against cataract formation in 50000 women. Similarly Robertson et al. found that intakes of vitamin C (300 mg/day) were associated with a 70% reduced risk of cataract [115].

Chapter IV

Prooxidant Mechanism of Vitamin C

Ascorbate is an excellent antioxidant. Despite the potential benefits of the administration of antioxidant vitamins on human health, some authors have raised questions on the potential side effects of the intake of large doses of these compounds. It is well established that most antioxidants, including vitamins, may promote free radical generation under certain circumstances, acting as prooxidant [20,116]). Administration of antioxidants can give protective effects or worsen damage, depending on where one is in the sequence of events (Figure 5) [58].

The *in vitro* prooxidant action of vitamin C is well-known. The initial reports of prooxidant effects of vitamin C *in vivo* were in 1998 [61,118]. Earlier studies of vitamin C at lower levels, 72 mg/day [119], reported only antioxidant effects but at higher amounts of vitamin C, 500 mg/day, there were possible prooxidant effects. The paradoxical behavior of vitamin C results because it is an excellent reducing agent. In addition to its well-known antioxidant properties, ascorbate, depending on the environment and conditions in which the molecule is active, can also act as a prooxidant [120].Mixtures of vitamin C and copper or iron have been used for decades to induce oxidative modifications of lipids, proteins and DNA (Wills, 1969). In nearly all the experimental systems where ascorbate has prooxidant properties, there is the simultaneous presence of redox active metals [121. The redox cycling of these metals is essential to the oxidation of vast majority of singlet state organic molecules.

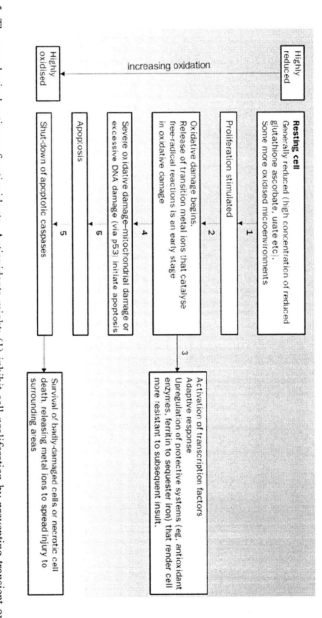

Figure 5. The paradoxical actions of antioxidants. Antioxidants might: (1) inhibit cell proliferation by preventing transient oxidations that stimulate protein phosphorylation and transcription factors; (2) protect against oxidative damage by scavenging excess reactive species, so blocking oxidation-dependent release of metal ions that catalyse free-radical damage; (3) prevent adaptation to oxidative damage by decreasing transcription-factor activation—eg, inhibition of myocardial ischaemic preconditioning; (4) accelerate oxidative damage by reducing transition-metal ions into their lower oxidation states that are better promoters of free-radical damage; and (5) inhibit free-radical-induced apoptosis, which might be either beneficial to the organism (in cell salvage) or deleterious (eg, if initiated cells do not die and lead to cancer development). Necrotic cell death might occur instead of apoptosis: necrosis releases cell contents (including transition metal ions) that spread the damage to surrounding areas [58].

Iron is an essential nutrient for normal cellular functions and has the capacity to accept and donate electrons, interconverting between the Fe^{3+} and Fe^{2+} forms. It is a useful component of cytochromes, oxygen-binding molecules (i.e., hemoglobin and myoglobin), and some enzymes. The iron-sulfur cluster and iron-protoporphyrin (i.e., heme) are cofactors of these enzymes. However, iron can also damage tissues by catalyzing the conversion of superoxide and hydrogen peroxide to free radical species that attack cellular membranes, proteins and DNA [122]. However, excess of iron can potentially generate oxidative stress via an increase in reactive oxygen species (ROS) production. Iron overload in humans and in experimental animals has been associated with oxidative stress [123-125]. In line with this, increased oxidative stress has been implicated in iron overload conditions and is thought to be due to iron-catalyzed generation of hydroxyl and alkoxyl radicals through Fenton chemistry [42].

In vitro induction of lipid peroxidation by ascorbate-iron systems is a standard test for inducing oxidative stress and testing antioxidant activity of other antioxidants. In this model system, chelation of Fe^{2+} by ascorbate creates an active catalyst for the production of ROS. When Fe^{3+} is present, vitamin C can convert Fe^{3+} into Fe^{2+}, which subsequently reacts with oxygen or hydrogen peroxide resulting in formation of superoxide anions and hydroxyl radicals (Figure 6) [126-128]. This paradoxical behavior results because it is an excellent reducing agent. As a reducing agent, it is able to reduce catalytic metals such as Fe^{3+} and Cu^{2+} to Fe^{2+} and Cu^{+} by following reactions:

1. $AH^{-} + Fe^{3+} \rightarrow A^{\bullet -} + Fe^{2+} + H^{+}$ ($k_2 \approx 10^2$ $M^{-1}s^{-1}$)
    $H_2O_2 + Fe^{2+} \rightarrow HO^{\bullet} + Fe^{3+} + HO^{-}$ ($k_2 = 76$ $M^{-1}s^{-1}$)
    $LOOH + Fe^{2+} \rightarrow LO^{\bullet} + Fe^{3+} + HO^{-}$ ($k_2 = 1.5 \times 10^3$ $M^{-1}s^{-1}$)
2. $AH^{-} + Cu^{2+} \rightarrow A^{\bullet -} + Cu^{+} + H^{+}$
    $H_2O_2 + Cu^{+} \rightarrow HO^{\bullet} + Cu^{2+} + HO^{-}$ ($k_2 = 4.7 \times 10^3$ $M^{-1}s^{-1}$)
    $LOOH + Cu^{+} \rightarrow LO^{\bullet} + Cu^{2+} + HO^{-}$ [8,20]

Fe^{2+} is oxidized to Fe^{3+} by the decomposition of lipid hydroperoxide (LOOH). The resulting accumulation of LOOH destroys membrane structure and function. The radical $HO^{\bullet}$ is very highly reactive and its estimated half-life in cells is only 10^{-9} seconds, and it can damage lipids, proteins, DNA, sugars, and generally all organic molecules [130]. Fe^{2+} is much more active than Fe^{3+} in decomposing hydroperoxide. Therefore, the rate of oxidation decreased as the oxidation proceeded and Fe^{2+} was oxidized to Fe^{3+}. In this case, the addition of ascorbic acid accelerated the oxidation, because it reduced Fe^{3+} to the more reactive Fe^{2+}. When Fe^{3+} was added initially, the oxidation proceeded quite slowly because it decomposed H_2O_2 only slowly. The addition of ascorbic acid again accelerated the oxidation. Thus, ascorbic acid can function as a prooxidant by reducing Fe^{3+} to Fe^{2+} [131].

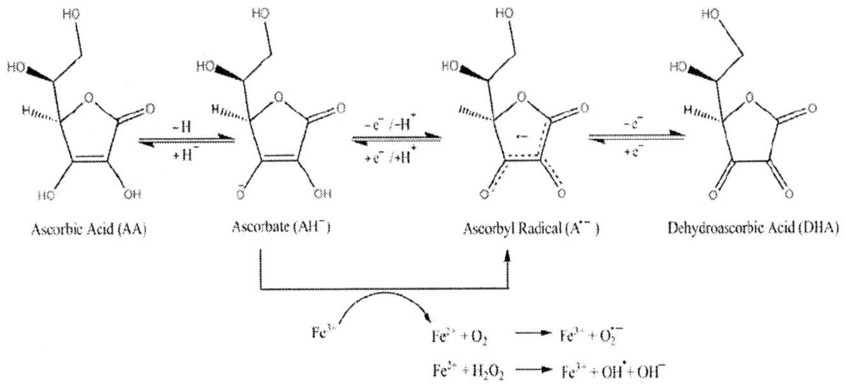

Figure 6. Prooxidant chemistry of ascorbic acid [129].

However, this vitamin C mediated Fenton reactions should be controlled in the human body due to efficient iron sequestration by metal binding proteins such as ferritin and transferrin. Iron ions circulate bound to plasma transferrin, and accumulate within cells in the form of ferritin. Under normal circumstances, only trace amounts of iron exist outside these physiologic sinks. In the healthy state there is never an appreciable concentration of 'free iron' (or iron chelated by low molecular weight compounds) [132,133]. Consequently, it has been argued that prooxidant effect may not be relevant *in vivo* [25,43]. On the other hand, vitamin C supplements have not been recommended for humans with high iron levels or in pathological conditions associated with iron overload such as thalassaemia or sickle cell disease. Because, vitamin C can mobilize such an enormous amount of iron from their high body iron stores to overwhelm the iron-binding capacity of iron-binding proteins, with the resultant free iron producing death within minutes to hours from iron-induced cardiac failure [134].

In vitro Studies Showing Prooxidant Effects of Vitamin C

Vitamin C protects against oxidation of isolated LDL by different types of oxidative stress, including metal ion dependent and independent processes [65]. In addition, *in vitro* studies have shown that physiological concentrations of ascorbic acid strongly inhibit LDL oxidation by vascular endothelial cells [135]. Despite the potential benefits of the administration of antioxidant vitamins on human health, some authors have raised questions on the potential side effects of the intake of large doses of these compounds [57]. It is well established that most antioxidants, including vitamins, may promote free radical generation under certain circumstances, acting as prooxidant. In fact, vitamin C, when incubated with LDL stored for certain time, and probably minimally oxidized, may promote their oxidation [136].

Vitamin C can induce chromosomal damage and cell death through generation of H_2O_2, especially in the presence of catalytic metals. Vitamin C can reduce or prevent H_2O_2-induced lipid peroxidation and the formation of OH-deoxyguanosine. It cannot therefore be assumed that vitamin C would always act as an antioxidant (Table 4). MacRae and Stich et al. [137] showed that freshly prepared ascorbate inhibited mitosis and induced chromosome aberrations in cultured Chinese hamster ovary cells. Fe(II) and Fe(III) (10^{-4} or 10^{-5} M) reduced or abolished the mitosis-inhibiting action of ascorbate. At 10^{-4} M, Fe(II) and Fe(III) strongly enhanced the chromosome-damaging capacity of ascorbate. Up to 100% of all examined metaphase plates had multiple chromosome exchanges or breaks. H_2O_2 and a H_2O_2:Fe(II) mixture (Fenton reagent) induced chromosome breaks and exchanges but to a lesser degree than did ascorbate: Cu(II), Mn(II), Fe(II), or Fe(III) mixtures. The authors concluded that the strong chromosome damaging capacity of ascorbate plus transition metals as seen in the *in vitro* test system poses a health hazard only properly designed *in vivo* studies can reveal. Zhao and Jung [138] suggested that ascorbic acid can cause strand breakage in DNA in the presence of oxygen and can initiate cell death in tissue culture, possibly through the generation of H_2O_2. Ascorbic acid incubated with Fe^{2+}-EDTA in the absence of H_2O_2, a deoxyribose degradation was observed, equivalent to about 20% of that produced when 0.85 mM H_2O_2 was present in the incubation medium. This result confirmed that ascorbic acid itself can produce $HO^{\bullet}$ radicals in the presence of Fe^{2+}-EDTA. Reactions of ascorbic acid with metals such as Fe^{2+} are thought to lead to the production of H_2O_2.

Bijur et al. [139] also examined the relationship between the anti- and prooxidant activities of ascorbic acid during oxidative stres by using the Chinese hamster ovary cell line AS52. The results of the study demonstrated that there were a temporal relationship between the antioxidant and prooxidant activities of ascorbic acid and oxidative stress. The antioxidative activity of ascorbic acid was directly related to its ability to reduce H_2O_2 formation in AS52 cells during oxidative stres. ascorbic acid (50 mM) functioned as an antioxidant, provided cells were treated with ascorbic acid prior to treatment with a radical generating system (RGS). That was demonstrated by a decrease in both the cytotoxic and mutagenic effects associated with treatment of AS52 cells with the RGS. Conversely, cotreatment of AS52 cells with the same concentration of ascorbic acid and the RGS resulted in an increase in the cytotoxic and mutagenic effects of oxidative stres when compared to cells treated with only the RGS, indicating that, under these conditions, ascorbic acid acts as a prooxidant.

Ascorbate can have both a protective and a prooxidant action in different membrane components under the same oxidative stress [140]. In fact, when incubated with iron, vitamin C is even used to propagate lipid peroxidation [134]. Laudicina and Marnett [141] showed that simultaneous addition of ascorbic acid and organic hydroperoxides to rat liver microsomes resulted in enhanced lipid peroxidation (approximately threefold) relative to incubation of organic hydroperoxides with microsomes alone. No lipid peroxidation was evident in incubations of ascorbate alone with microsomes. The results reveal a synergistic prooxidant effect of ascorbic acid on hydroperoxide-dependent lipid peroxidation.

Likewise, Yen et al. [142] were investigated the antioxidant and prooxidant properties of ascorbic acid by using deoxyribose assay, scavenging of free radicals and chelation of Fe^{2+}; and effects on oxidative DNA damage to human lymphocytes using single cell gel electrophoresis. ascorbic acid accelerate the oxidation of deoxyribose induced by Fe^{3+}–EDTAJH$_2$O$_2$. Ascorbic acid causes strand breakage in DNA in the presence of oxygen and can induce cell death in tissue culture, possibly through the generation of H_2O_2. The authors suggested that a marked reducing ability and a weak metal-chelating effect of ascorbic acid might cause the pro-oxidant action of ascorbic acid. Sahu and Washington [143] performed a study to determine the extent of nuclear DNA degradation induced by iron, iron-ascorbate, or iron-bleomycin under aerobic conditions in a model system using isolated rat liver nuclei. Iron induced concentration-dependent DNA degradation, and this effect was enhanced by ascorbate and bleomycin. The antioxidants catalase, dimethyl sulfoxide, and diallyl sulfide significantly reduced the iron-ascorbate-induced DNA damage, whereas superoxide dismutase and dimethyl sulfoxide significantly reduced iron-bleomycin-induced damage. Glutathione significantly increased the iron-bleomycin-induced DNA damage. These results suggest that the reactive oxygen species generated by iron, iron-ascorbate, and iron-bleomycin are responsible for the DNA strand breaks in isolated rat liver nuclei.

Zhang and Omaye [144] investigated the antioxidant and prooxidant effects of β-carotene, α-tocopherol and ascorbic acid on human lung cells at different oxygen (O_2) tensions. Free radical initiator, 2,2'-azobis (2-amidinopropane) dihydrochloride (AAPH), was used to induce the cellular damage associated with lipid peroxidation, protein oxidation and DNA breaks. The antioxidant effects of alpha-tocopherol, ascorbic acid, and mixtures of the three antioxidant compounds also were reduced by the high O_2 conditions.

Higher concentrations of vitamin C induce apoptotic cell death in various tumor cell lines including oral squamous cell carcinoma and salivary gland tumor cell lines, possibly via its prooxidant action [144]. Akatov et al. [146] investigated the effect of cobalt octa-4,5-carboxyphthalocyanine propylenglycol ether (ETp)+ascorbic acid combination on apoptotic death of tumor cells. ETp proposed for antitumor therapy potentiates the cytotoxic effect of ascorbate on HL-60 human leukemia cells. Combination of these substances caused the formation of H_2O_2 in the medium and initiated apoptotic death of cells. Addition of ETp+ scorbic acid to cells caused a cytotoxic effect, while ETp or ascorbic acid alone were nontoxic for HL-60 cells, which attests to synergic effect of the system components.

De Laurenzi et al. [147] showed that human neuroectodermal cells exposed to H_2O_2 or ascorbate die by programmed cell death induced by oxidative stress. The cell death by H_2O_2 occurs within 4 h and involves approximately 80% of B-mel melanoma cells, while ascorbate causes cell death of approximately 86% of B-mel cells within 24 h. The cell death observed in the study suggested a pro-oxidant, rather than anti-oxidant, role for ascorbic acid at physiological concentrations under these experimental conditions.

Lefebvre and Pezerat [148] were investigated the reactions of various chromate pigments and ascorbate by an ESR spin trapping technique. Production of Cr(V) was detected directly and productions of very electrophilic reactive oxygen species (ROS) was detected via the oxidation of formate. The reaction of ascorbate with various chromate pigments produces ROS as evidenced by formate oxidation in aqueous solution at 37°C.

Park and Lee [149] examined the effect of ascorbic acid on reperfusion injury after hepatic cold preservation. The portal pressure, lactate dehydrogenase and purine nucleoside phosphorylase activities were elevated by cold ischemia/reperfusion and these changes were augmented at a concentration of 2 mM ascorbic acid. Cold ischemia/reperfusion decreased the reduced to oxidized glutathione ratio, whereas it increased the level of lipid peroxidation and mitochondrial swelling. But were augmented at 2 mM ascorbic acid. The authors suggest that cold ischemia/reperfusion injury is associated with a higher level of oxidative stress and ascorbic acid may act not only as an antioxidant but also as a prooxidant during cold ischemia/reperfusion.

Table 4. Summary of *in vitro* studies indicates prooxidant effect of ascorbic acid

Study system	Purpose	Effects of Ascorbic acid	Reference
Chinese hamster ovary cells	Incubation cells with ascorbic acid, Cu(II), Mn(II) and Fe(II) and Fe(III)	Freshly prepared ascorbate inhibited mitosis and induced chromosome aberrations.	137
Chinese hamster ovary cell line AS52.	cotreatment of AS52 cells with the same concentration of AA and the RGS	Cotreatment of cells with AA and the RGS results in an increase in the cytotoxic and mutagenic effects of oxidative stres when compared to cells treated with only the RGS	139
Rat liver microsomes	effects of ascorbic acid and organic hydroperoxides on lipid peroxidation	Simultaneous addition of ascorbic acid and organic hydroperoxides to rat liver microsomes resulted in enhanced lipid peroxidation relative to incubation of organic hydroperoxides with microsomes alone indicating a synergistic prooxidant effect of ascorbic acid on hydroperoxide-dependent lipid peroxidation.	141
Human lymphocytes	investigated the antioxidant and prooxidant properties of ascorbic acid by using deoxyribose assay	AA at a concentration of 1.65 mM, accelerate the oxidation of deoxyribose induced by Fe^{3+}—EDTAJH$_2$O$_2$. AA causes strand breakage in DNA in the presence of oxygen possibly through the generation of hydrogen peroxide	142
HL–60 human leukemia cells	effect of ETp+Asc combination on apoptotic death of tumor cells.	Combination of ETp+Asc caused the formation of H$_2$O$_2$ in the medium and initiated apoptotic death of cells. Addition of 5 μM ETp and 100 μM Asc to cells caused a cytotoxic effect.	146
Human neuroectodermal cells	exposed to 1–5 mM hydrogen peroxide or 10 nM-1 mM ascorbate	Cells died by programmed cell death induced by oxidative stres suggesting a pro-oxidant role for ascorbic acid	147
Cell culture medium	effect of solubility of different chromate pigments and ascorbate on the production of ROS	Increased production of reactive oxygen species (ROS)	148
Cold ischemia/reperfusion model of liver	effect of ascorbic acid on reperfusion injury after hepatic cold preservation	Cold ischemia/reperfusion injury is associated with a higher level of oxidative stress and ascorbic acid may act not only as an antioxidant but also as a prooxidant during cold ischemia/reperfusion.	149

Chapter V

In vivo Studies Showing Prooxidant Effects of Vitamin C

There is a lot of studies showing *in vivo* antioxidant effect of vitamin C against different chemical induced oxidative damage (Table 5). In the study by Gipp et al. [150], the influence of high levels of dietary Fe and ascorbic acid on the deleterious effects of 250 ppm dietary Cu was investigated. ascorbic acid had no effect on altering the level of Fe retained in the liver or intestine of pigs, but did increase the plasma Fe level, the degree of saturation of plasma transferrin, and the rate of removal from plasma and uptake by RBC of Fe. It is concluded that the Fe deficiency induced by high dietary Cu is due to impairment in Fe absorption from the gastrointestinal tract and that this impairment is ameliorated by ascorbic acid. Suzuki and Yoshida [151] were studied the protective and therapeutic effects of surplus dietary iron and ascorbic acid on cadmium toxicity in rats and the effect of surplus iron and ascorbic acid on lead toxicity. Supplementation of 400 ppm of iron and 1% of ascorbic acid to the lead containing diet prevented the growth depression and anemia and caused reductions of concentrations of lead in the kidney and tibia. Recoveries from the growth retardation and anemia were not observed in rats within a week after the transfer to the non-lead diet with or without iron and ascorbic acid. These results suggest that iron prevents the growth depression and anemia in rats ingesting lead by an inhibition of lead absorption. Also, Erdoğan et al. [152] were investigated the effects of cadmium on performance, antioxidant defense system, liver and kidney functions, and cadmium accumulation in selected tissues of broiler chickens and whether ascorbic acid would reverse the possible adverse effects of cadmium. However, ascorbic acid did not ameliorate the growth inhibitory effect of cadmium nor did it prevent accumulation of cadmium in analyzed tissues.

Kang et al. [153] reported the dual role of vitamin C on paraquat-induced lung injury, which appears to depend on the metal ions released from damaged cells. They investigated the effect of vitamin C on paraquat-induced lung damage in rats. Vitamin C (10 mg/kg) given at the time when the extensive tissue damage was in progress aggravated the oxidative damage, while it protected against the damage when given before the initiation of the damage. The authors concluded that vitamin C can either aggravate or alleviate the oxidative tissue damage depending on the presence of metal ions released from damaged cells.

In a recent report, it has been demonstrated that large doses of exogenous iron (200 mg) and ascorbic acid (75 mg) promote the release of iron from iron binding proteins and also enhance *in vitro* lipid peroxidation in serum of guinea pigs [123]. The iron-loaded animals fed the low ascorbate dose had decreased plasma alpha-tocopherol levels and increased plasma levels of triglycerides and $F_{(2)}$-isoprostanes, specific and sensitive markers of *in vivo* lipid peroxidation. In contrast, the two groups of animals fed the high ascorbate dose had significantly lower hepatic $F_{(2)}$-isoprostane levels than the groups fed the low ascorbate dose, irrespective of iron load. These data indicated that the combination of iron loading with a low ascorbate status caused additional pathophysiological changes, in particular, increased plasma triglycerides. This finding supports the hypothesis that high intake of iron along with ascorbic acid could increase *in vivo* lipid peroxidation of LDL and therefore could increase risk of atheroscerosis.

Takahashi [154] fed male Jcl:SD rats a laboratory ration for 1 week and then an experimental diet containing 5% ascorbic acid. Dead rats and those killed were necropsied and hemorrhagic foci were counted. Diarrhea was observed in the treated rats throughout the experiment. Ascorbic acid did not have a hemorrhagic effect. At necropsy, edema of the stomach, hypertrophy of the kidneys and enlargement of the cecum were found in 2/6, 1/6, and 6/6 rats, respectively.

Premkumar and Bowlus [155] investigated whether ascorbic acid and iron co-supplementation in ascorbic acid-sufficient mice increased hepatic oxidative stress. C3H/He mice were fed diets supplemented with iron to 100 mg/kg diet or 300 mg/kg diet with or without ascorbic acid (15 g/kg diet) for 3 wk. Ascorbic acid increased MDA but only in mice fed the low-iron diet. The high-iron diet reduced GPx, CAT, SOD, and GST activities regardless of ascorbic acid supplementation. In contrast, ascorbic acid reduced GPx and CAT activities only in mice fed the low-iron diet. These results of the study suggested that ascorbic acid supplementation can have prooxidant effects in the liver. However, ascorbic acid did not further increase the oxidative stress induced by increased dietary iron.

The study by Chatterjee [156] was carried out on the effects of subacute rubidium chloride toxicity in rats in relation to L -ascorbic acid metabolism and certain enzymes of liver, kidney, and brain tissues as well as hepatic lipid composition. Rubidium-treated (ip) rats showed drastic decrease in growth along with a severe anemic condition which could not be reversed by oral L-ascorbic acid supplementation. Rubidium toxicity markedly disturbed the normal histological pattern of both liver and kidney cells and also significantly changed the hepatic lipid composition. Brain tissue was found to be affected severely as showed by certain enzyme activity alterations. L-Ascorbic acid supplementation to the treated group of animals could afford some protection against the alterations of certain liver enzymes as well as in regard to the histological changes of either liver and kidney as caused by rubidium toxicity.

Elhaïmeur et al. [157] investigated the effects of a vitamin C supplemented diet on blood pressure, body and liver weights, liver antioxidant status, iron and copper levels were investigated in DOCA-salt treated and untreated Sprague-Dawley (SD) male rats after 8 weeks of treatment. Vitamin C supplementation did not affect the overall antioxidant defenses of control SD rat livers. In contrast, vitamin C supplementation accentuated the DOCA-salt induced accumulation of liver iron and lipid peroxidation. The authors suggested that DOCA-salt treatment induces an accumulation of iron in rat livers which is responsible for the prooxidant effect of vitamin C.

Nowak et al. [158] explored whether ip administration of ascorbic acid in a dose of 500 mg/kg, once a day for 3 following days, affected the content of lipid peroxidation products: malondialdehyde (MDA) and conjugated dienes (CD) in organs of mice. Injection of ascorbic acid caused 2.1-, 1.3- and 1.8-fold increase in the concentration of this vitamin in liver, spleen and lungs, respectively, while the content of MDA and CD in these organs did not differ from values found in animals treated with 0.9% NaCl. The authors suggested that this animal model ascorbic acid did not act as a prooxidant enhancing the lipid peroxidation in various tissues.

An increase in oxidative stress may contribute to the development of diabetic complications. Therefore, Young et al. [159] investigated the effects of ascorbate supplementation on oxidative stress in the streptozotocin diabetic rat. In this study, markers of lipid peroxidation (malondialdehyde [MDA] and diene conjugates) were increased in plasma and erythrocytes of untreated diabetic animals, and levels of the antioxidants ascorbate and retinol were reduced. Insulin treatment normalized MDA and ascorbate levels, although ascorbate metabolism remained disturbed, as indicated by increased levels of dehydroascorbate. High-dose ascorbate supplementation in the absence of insulin treatment restored plasma ascorbate to normal levels. The author concluded that high-dose ascorbate supplementation should be approached with caution in diabetes, as ascorbate may exert both antioxidant and prooxidant effects *in vivo*.

In the study by Speit et al. [160], vitamin C ranged from 200 to 10 000 mg/kg body weight was administered orally as well as by intraperitoneal injection to Chinese hamsters. Sulfhydryl compounds such as cysteine and glutathione inhibited the SCE induction by vitamin C *in vitro* owing to their reducing capacity. The results were discussed with regard to the primary damage that may lead to an induction of sister-chromatid exchanges (SCEs) by ascorbate, and the possible mutagenic danger to humans posed by vitamin C. Ascorbate also caused a dose-dependent increase in SCEs in Chinese hamster ovary (CHO) cells and in human lymphocytes. Moreover, in the DNA synthesis inhibition test with HeLa cells, ascorbate gave results typical of DNA-damaging chemicals [161].

Besides bisphenol A (BPA), nonylphenol (NP) and octylphenol (OP) inherent effects on endocrine system, they are also known to inflict oxidative stress by affecting the redox status in the exposed organs [162,163]. Aydoğan et al. [164] performed a study to investigate whether these estrogenic chemicals, BPA, NP and octylphenol OP, induce oxidative stress in reproductive tract of male rats and co-administration of vitamin C can prevent any possible oxidative stress. Wistar male rats were divided were administered BPA, NP and OP orally thrice a week for 45 days or vitamin C (60 mg/kg/day) were administered orally along with BPA, OP and NP (25 mg/kg/day) treatments. Histological examination showed that vitamin C co-administrated groups had much more congestion areas, atrophy and germinal cell debris in testes than those observed in other groups. Abnormal sperm percentages of BPA, BPA+C, NP+C and OP+C groups were increased. The results of this study demonstrated that BPA, NP and OP generate reactive oxygen species that cause oxidative damage in testes of rats.

Appenroth et al. [165] investigated the influence of high dose ascorbic acid (5 g/kg body weight) on chromate (Cr, 10 mg/kg) induced proteinuria, which is a sensitive parameter of its nephrotoxicity, was investigated in adult female Wistar rats. Proteinuria was completely prevented by enhancement of extracellular reduction of Cr(VI) to Cr(III) followed by rapid renal excretion when Cr and ascorbic acid were given concomitantly. With an interval up to 1 h between Cr and ascorbic acid, proteinuria was decreased probably by the radical scavenging function of ascorbic acid. At an interval of 3 h ascorbic acid enhanced Cr toxicity by increased intracellular Cr reduction. If the interval was increased to 5 h or if Cr was given 24 h after ascorbic acid, no influence of ascorbic acid could be detected. The authors suggests that ascorbic acid is a very effective reductant of Cr which can influence Cr nephrotoxicity in very high concentrations. It depends on the interval between Cr and ascorbic acid administration whether or not there is a beneficial effect of ascorbic acid in Cr nephrotoxicity.

In slices prepared from cerebral cortex of rats receiving high doses of vitamin C, Song et al. [166] reported increased TBARS in a dose-dependent manner. Likewise, Aydoğan et al. [167] investigated the oxidative effects of BPA, NP and OP on the brain tissue of male rats and if coadministration of vitamin C, an antioxidant, can prevent any possible oxidative stress. Decreased levels of reduced glutathione (GSH) were found in the brains of BPA, NP, OP treated rats. The end product of lipid peroxidation, malondialdehyde (MDA), appeared at significantly higher concentrations in the BPA, NP, and OP treated groups. In histopathologic examination, the vitamin C co-administrated groups had much more hyperchromatic cells in the brain cortex than that observed in the groups treated with only BPA, NP, and OP. Further, the results of our previous study demonstrate that BPA, NP and OP generate reactive oxygen species that caused oxidative damage in the brain of male rats [168]. In the kidney tissue, the highest lactate dehydrogenase (LDH) activity was present in BPA+C, NP+C and OP+C groups compared to BPA, NP, and OP groups. The malondialdehyde (MDA) levels were significantly higher while glutathione (GSH) levels were lower in treatment groups than controls. Furthermore, an increase was observed in MDA levels whereas a decrease was observed in GSH levels in BPA+C, NP+C and OP+C groups compared to BPA, NP and OP groups, respectively. These finding were in accordance with immunohistochemical staining of MDA and GSH. Histopathological examination of the kidneys of rats in BPA, OP, NP, BPA+C, NP+C and OP+C groups revealed necrotic lesions, congestion and mononuclear cell infiltration. In conclusion BPA, NP and OP might induce oxidative damage in kidney of rats. Thus, co-administration of vitamin C with BPA, NP and OP to male rats augments this damage in the kidney, brain and reproductive system of male rats.

Table 5. Summary of *in vivo* studies indicate prooxidant effect of ascorbic acid

Study system	Purpose	Effects of Ascorbic acid	Reference
Guinea pigs	the iron-loaded animals fed with ascorbic acid	high intake of iron along with ascorbic acid could increase *in vivo* lipid peroxidation of LDL and therefore could increase risk of atheroscerosis	123
Rat	the effect of vitamin C on paraquat-induced lung damage	vitamin C can either aggravate or alleviate the oxidative tissue damage depending on the presence of metal ions released from damaged cells.	153
Jcl:SD rats	Fed with %5 ascorbic acid containing food	Diarrhea was observed in the treated rats. Edema of the stomach, hypertrophy of the kidneys and enlargement of the cecum were found in 2/6, 1/6, and 6/6 rats.	154
C3H/He mice	effects of ascorbic acid and iron co-supplementation in ascorbic acid-sufficient mice on hepatic oxidative stress	Ascorbic acid increased MDA but only in mice fed the low-iron diet. Ascorbic acid reduced GPx and CAT activities only in mice fed the low-iron diet	155
Rat	effects on subacute rubidium chloride toxicity	Rubidium-treated (ip) rats showed drastic decrease in growth along with a severe anemic condition which could not be reversed by oral L-ascorbic acid supplementation.	156
Sprague-Dawley (SD) male rat	effects of a vitamin C supplemented diet on DOCA-salt treated and untreated Sprague-Dawley male rats	Vitamin C supplementation accentuated the DOCA-salt induced accumulation of liver iron and lipid peroxidation. DOCA-salt treatment induces an accumulation of iron in rat livers which is responsible for the prooxidant effect of vitamin C	157
Chinese hamsters	effects of vitamin C administered orally and by intraperitoneal injection on the induction of sister-chromatid exchanges (SCE)	Vitamin C did not produce an increment in the basal frequency of SCE.	160
Female Wistar rat	the influence of ascorbic acid (AA, 5 g/kg body weight) on chromate (Cr, 10 mg/kg) induced proteinuria	Proteinuria was completely prevented when Cr and AA were given concomitantly. If the interval was increased to 5 h or if Cr was given 24 h after AA, no influence of AA could be detected.	165

Chapter VI

Human Studies Showing Prooxidant Effects of Vitamin C

In 1998, the most interesting paper about prooxidant role of vitamin C published in Nature. Podmore et al. [61] supplemented 30 healthy volunteers (16 females and 14 males aged between 17 and 49) with 500 mg of vitamin C daily for 6 wk following 3 wk each of baseline and placebo periods. The plasma concentration of vitamin C was elevated by 60% after vitamin C supplementation. The levels of oxidized DNA bases [8-oxogua and 8-oxoadenine (8-oxoade)], were measured in peripheral blood lymphocytes using GC-MS. The baseline levels of 8-oxogua and 8-oxoade were reported to be 30 and 8 lesions per 105 unoxidized bases, respectively. After vitamin C supplementation, 8-oxogua levels were significantly reduced relative to baseline and placebo, whereas the levels of 8-oxoade were significantly elevated. The reduced 8-oxogua and the elevated 8-oxoade levels returned to baseline levels after a vitamin C washout period of 7 wk.

Cooke et al. reported possible prooxidant effects of vitamin C at intakes of roughly 400 and 500 mg per day [118,169]. In healthy patients, but at oxidative risk, the prooxidant effects of high doses of vitamin C have also been reported. In athletes with muscle injury and thus in inflammatory situation, 12.5 mg of vitamin C/kg body weight resulted in increased lipid peroxidation [170].

EDTA chelation therapy is an often used treatment aimed at reducing calcium deposits, removing heavy metals, controlling lipid peroxidation resulting from free radical pathology, and reducing platelet aggregation in the clinical management of atherosclerosis and related disorders. Chelation therapy is thought to not only to remove contaminating metals but also to decrease free radical production [171]. Moreover, in chelation therapy, high doses of vitamin C are often used as an adjuvant of the treatment [172]. Vitamin C is a known antioxidant but at the high levels (5 g, intravenous) often used during chelation therapy its effects have not been ascertained. In this setting, its use may be beneficial as an antioxidant or deleterious as high doses of ascorbate can have prooxidant effects, especially in the presence of elevated amounts of transition metals [8,173]. Since EDTA chelation therapy is proposed to not only remove metals but also have antioxidant properties [171], it has been used in the treatment of these diseases. The standard EDTA cocktail contains high doses of sodium ascorbate (5 g). The health benefits of vitamin C are the subject of debate and the potential danger of megadoses of vitamin C has been reviewed [174]. Hininger et al. [175] designed a study to determine if the vitamin C added to standard chelation therapy cocktails was prooxidant. They administered a standard EDTA cocktail solution with or without 5 g of sodium ascorbate. One hour following the standard chelation therapy, there were highly significant prooxidant effects on lipids, proteins, and DNA associated with decreased activities of RBC glutathione peroxidase and superoxide dismutase while in the absence of sodium ascorbate, there were no acute signs of oxidative damage They observed a higher rate of disulfide formation in patients receiving the EDTA cocktail with vitamin C. The decrease in plasma SH groups is known to be induced by a wide array of ROS and is one of the most immediate responses to an elevation in the level of oxidative stress.

Chen et al. [176] hypothesize that adjuvant therapy with larger doses of ascorbic acid in hemodialysis patients with iron overload may raise the risk of increasing free radical generation. The oxidative stress of intravenous ascorbic acid supplementation in hemodialysis patients was evaluated in this study. Six healthy subjects and 29 hemodialysis patients were enrolled. Chemical scavenging activity of various compounds was measured by in vitro 2,2-diphenyl-1-picrylhydrazyl (DPPH) assay. Free radical generation was determined in vitro by lucigenin-enhanced chemiluminescence (LucCL) assay on blood samples. Blood biochemistries were also measured simultaneously in hemodialysis patients 1 minute before and 5 minutes later in the presence or absence of intravenous injection of 300 mg ascorbic acid. Ascorbic acid presented a strong antioxidant effect in DPPH chemical reaction. On the contrary, it exerted pro-oxidant effect when mixed with plasma or whole blood of healthy subjects and hemodialysis patients. The pro-oxidant effect of ascorbic acid detected by LucCL was attenuated by various iron chelators and superoxide dismutase. In hemodialysis patients, the changes of LucCL intensity were significantly higher in the ascorbic acid-treated group than those in the control group. Persons with excess ascorbic acid supplement in the blood or plasma generate iron-chelator-suppressible chemiluminescents suggestive of free radical formation.

Lachili et al. [177] investigated the effect of a daily combined iron supplementation (100 mg/d as fumarate) and vitamin C (500 mg/d as ascorbate) for the third trimester of pregnancy on lipid peroxidation (plasma TBARS), antioxidant micronutriments (Zn, Se, retinol, vitamin E, (β-carotene) and antioxidant metalloenzymes (RBC Cu-Zn SOD and Se-GPX). The iron-supplemented group (n=27) was compared to a control group (n=27), age and number of pregnancies matched. At delivery, all the women exhibited normal Hb and ferritin values. In the supplemented group, plasma iron level was higher than in the control group (26.90 ± 5.52 mmol/L) and TBARs plasma levels were significantly enhanced (3.62 ± 0.36 vs 3.01 ± 0.37 mmol/L). These data show that pharmalogical doses of iron, associated with high vitamin C intakes, can result in uncontrolled lipid peroxidation. This is predictive of adverse effects for the mother and the fetus. This study illustrates the potential harmful effects of iron supplementation when prescribed only on the assumption of anemia and not on the bases of biological criteria.

Chapter VII

Conclusion

Vitamin C is one of the important and essential vitamins for human health. It is required for the optimal activity of several important biosynthetic enzymes and is therefore essential for various metabolic pathways in the body. Also Vitamin C, which known as an antioxidant *in vitro* and *in vivo*, very effectively protects biomolecules in human cells against peroxidative damage by scavenging oxygen-derived free radicals and by regenerating vitamin E from its' radical form. Ascorbic acid is located in the extracellular and hydrophilic regions of the cell. Ascorbic acid, in the extracellular matrix, is the antioxidant that first defends cells. Antioxidant protection involves a variety of factors, i.e. concentration of antioxidant compounds, O_2 tensions, and interactions among the antioxidant compounds. Likewise, we can expect that the outcome of *in vitro* study is different from that of *in vivo* due to even more complicated biological systems. Base on the numerous biochemical, clinical and epidemiological studies suggest that, vitamin C supplementation reduces risk of some diseases such as heart diseases, cancer, atherosclerosis in mammals and human.

Paradoxically, vitamin C, can also act as a prooxidant depending on the environment and conditions in which the molecule is active. A majority of the studies *in vitro* and *in vivo* is addressed the interaction of vitamin C with iron showing either no effect or prooxidant effect of vitamin C. Ascorbate and the ascorbyl radical can autoxidize in the presence of redox active transition metal ions such as copper and iron ions and yield hydroxl radicals.

The authors reviewed selected articles from the literature to encourage and stimulate further interest and investigation into the usefulness of vitamin C.

Future studies may elucidate specific roles and mechanism of antioxidant and/or prooxidant action of vitamins C in health and disease.

References

[1]   McCord, CP. Scurvy as an occupational disease, VII Scurvy in the world's army. *Journal of Occupational Medicine,* 1971 13, 586-592.

[2]   Svent-Gyorgi, A. On the function of hexuronic acid in the respiration of the cabbage leaf. *Journal of Biological Chemistry,* 1931 90,385-393.

[3]   Reichstein, T; Grussner, A; Oppenauer, R. Synthese der L-ascobinsaüre (C-vitamin). *Helv. Chim. Acta,* 1933 16, 1019-1033.

[4]   Nishikimi, M; Yagi, K. Biochemistry and molecular biology of ascorbic acid biosynthesis. In: Haris RJ, editor. *Subcellular Biochemistry.* New York: Plenum Pres; 1996; 17.

[5]   Jaffe, GM. Ascorbic acid, in Encyclopedia of Chemical Technology. 3rd Edition. John Wiley & Sons; 1984.

[6]   Duarte, TL; Lunec, J. "Review: When is an antioxidant not an antioxidant? A review of novel actions and reactions of vitamin C". *Free Radical Research,* 2005 39 (7), 671–686.

[7]   Buettner, GR. The pecking order of free radicals and antioxidants: lipid peroxidation, α-tocopherol, and ascorbate. Archieves of Biochemistry and. *Biophyscics,* 1993 30, 535–543.

[8]   Buettner, GR; Jurkiewicz, BA. Catalytic metals, ascorbate and free radicals: combinations to avoid. *Radiation Research,* 1996 145, 532–541.

[9]   Chatterjee, IB; Chatterjee, GC; Ghosh, NC; Ghosh, JJ; Guha BC. Biological synthesis of L-ascorbic acid in animal tissues: conversion of L-gulonolactone into L-ascorbic acid. *Biochem. Journal,* 1960 74(1), 193–203.

[10]   Ray Chaudhuri, C; Chatterjee, IB. L-Ascorbic Acid Synthesis in Birds: *Phylogenetic Trend. Science,* 1969 164, 435-436.

[11] Arrigon, IO. Ascorbate system in plant development. *Journal of Bioenergy Biomembrane, 1994* 6(4), 407–419.

[12] Nishikimi, M; Kawai, T; Yagi, K. Guinea pigs possess a highly mutated gene for L-gulono-g-lactone oxidase, as key enzyme for L-ascorbic acid biosynthesis missing in this species. *Journal of Biological Chemistry,* 1992 267, 21967-21972.

[13] Nishikimi, M; Fukuyama, R; Minoshima, S; Shimizu, S; Shimizu, N; Yagi, K. Cloning and chromosomal mapping of the human nonfunctional gene for L-gulono-g-lactone oxidase, the enzyme for L-ascorbic acid biosynthesis missing in man. *Journal of Biological Chemistry,* 1994 269, 13685-13688.

[14] Tsukaguchi, H; Tokui, T; Mackenzie, B; Berger, UV; Chen, X Z; Wang, YX. A family of mammalian Na+-dependent L-ascorbic acid transporters. *Nature,* 1999 399, 70−75.

[15] Nandi, A; Mukhopadhyay, CK; Ghosh, MK; Chattopadhyay, DJ; Chatterjee, IB. Evolutionary significance of vitamin C biosynthesis in terrestrial vertebrates. *Free Radical Biology and Medicine,* 1997 22 (6), 1047-1054.

[16] Hellman, L; Burns, JJ. Metabolism of L-ascorbic acid-1-C14 in man. *Journal of Biological Chemistry*, 1958 230, 923-930.

[17] Hunt, JV. Ascorbic acid and diabetus mellitus. In: Harris, RJ, editor, *Subcellular Biochemistry,* Vol: 25. New York: Plenum Pres; 1995; 369.

[18] Kallner, A; Horing, D; Hartman D. Kinteics of ascorbic acid in humans. In: Seib PA, editor. Ascorbic acid: Chemistry, metabolism and uses Tolbert BM. Advances in Chemistry Series No.200. Washington DC: American Chemical Society; 1982; 385-400.

[19] Johnson, CS. Biomarkers for establishing a tolerable upper intake level for vitamin C. *Nutrition Reviewes,* 1999 57, 71-77.

[20] Halliwell, B; Gutteridge, JMC. Free radicals in biology and medicine, 3rd Edition. Oxford: Oxford University Press; 1999.

[21] Food and Nutrition Board, U.S. National Research Council- National Academy of Sciences Recommended Dietary Allowance, National Academy of Sciences, Washington D.C.; 1974.

[22] Food and Nutrition Board and Panel on Dietary Antioxidants and Related Compounds Vitamin C, 2000.

[23] Levine M; Wang, Y; Padayatty, SJ; Morrow, J. A new recommended dietary allowance of vitamin C for healthy young women. *PNAS,* 2001 98, 9842- 9846.

[24] Bendich, A; Langseth, L. Safety of vitamin A. *American Journal of Clinical Nutrition,* 1989 49,358-371.

[25] Carr, AC; Frei, B. Does vitamin C act as pro-oxidant under physiological conditions? *FASEB J,* 1999 13, 1007-1024.

[26] Dawes, MB; Austin, J; Partridge, DA. Inorganic and analytical aspects of vitamin C chemistry. In: Dawes MB; Austin J; Partridge DA, editors. *Vitamin C its Chemistry and Biochemistry.* Cambridge: Royal Society of Chemistry; 1991; 115-146.

[27] Mapson, LW. Vitamins in fruits. In: Hulme EC, editor. *The Biochemistry of Fruits and their Products.* London: Academic Press; 1970; 369-383.

[28] Johnson, CS; Steinberg, FM; Rucker, RB. Ascorbic acid. In: Rucker RB; Sultie JW; McCormick, DB; Machlin LJ., editor. *Handbook of Vitamins.* New York: Marcel Dekker Inc; 1998; 529-585.

[29] Levine, M; Rumsey, SC; Wang, Y; Park, JB; Daruwala, R. Vitamin C. In Stipanuk MH, editor. Biochemical and Physiological Aspects of Human Nutrition. Philadelphia: W B Saunders; 2000; 541–567.

[30] Levine, M; Hartzell, W. Ascorbic acid: the concept of optimum requirements. Annual New York Academy of Science, 1987 498, 424-444.

[31] Jung, CH; Wells, WW. Ascorbic acid is a stimulatory cofactor for mitochondrial glycerol-3-phosphate dehydrogenase. *Biochem. Biophys. Res. Comm.,* 1997 239 457-462.

[32] Levine, M. New concepts in the biology and biochemistry of ascorbic acid. *New England Journal of Medicine,* 1986 31, 892-902.

[33] Phillips, CL; Yeowell, HN. Vitamin C, collagen biosynthesis, and aging. In: Packer L, Fuchs J, editors. Vitamin C in health and disease. New York: Marcel Dekker Inc; 1997; 205–230.

[34] Hulse, JD; Ellis, SR; Henderson, LM. Carnitine biosynthesis-beta hydroxylation of trimethyllysine by an α-keto glutarate dependent mitochondrial dioxygenase. *Journal of Biological Chemistry,* 1978 253,1654-1659.

[35] Kaufman, S. Dopamine-beta-hydroxylase. *Journal of Psychiatric Research,* 1974 11, 303–316.

[36] Ginter, E; Bobek, P; Jurcovicova, M. Role of ascorbic acid in lipid metabolism. In: Seith, PA; Toblert, BM, editors. Ascorbic acid, chemistry, metabolism and uses. Washington D.C: American Chemical Society; 1982; 381-393.

[37] Hallberg, L; Brune, M; Rossander-Hulthen, L. Is there a physiological role of vitamin C in iron absorption? Annual New York Academy of Science, 1987 498, 324–332.

[38] Bucala, R. Lipid and lipoprotein oxidation: basic mechanisms and unresolved questions in vivo. *Redox Report,* 1996 2, 291–307.

[39] Ho, YS; Magnenat, JL; Gargano, M; Cao J. The nature of antioxidant defense mechanisms: A lesson from transgenic studies. *Environmental Health Perspectives,* 1998 106, 1219–1228.

[40] Halliwell B. Reactive oxygen species in living systems: Source, biochemistry and role in human disease. *American Journal of Medicine,* 1991 91, 14–22.

[41] Ames, BN; Shigenaga, MK; Hagen, TM. Oxidants, antioxidants, and the degenerative diseases of aging. *Proceeding of the National Academy of Science U.S.A.,* 1993 90, 7915–22.

[42] Halliwell B. Antioxidants in human health and disease. *Annual Reviews of Nutrition,* 1996 16, 33–50.

[43] Halliwell, B. Antioxidant defence mechanism: From the beginning to the end (of the beginning). *Free Radical Research,* 1999 31, 261– 272.

[44] Noiri, E; Nakao, A; Uchida K. Oxidative and nitrosative stress in acute renal ischemia. *American Journal of Physiolology: Renal Physiology,* 2001 281, F948–F957.

[45] Marnett, LJ. Oxyradicals and DNA damages. *Carcinogenesis.* 2000 21, 361–370.

[46] Ozcan, A; Sacar, M; Aybek, H. The effects of iloprost and vitamin C on kidney as a remote organ after ischemia/ reperfusion of lower extremities. *Journal of Surgical Research,* 2006 140 (1), 20–26.

[47] Berlett, BS; Stadtman ER. Protein oxidation in aging, disease, and oxidative stress. *Journal of Biological Chemistry,* 1997 272, 20313–20316.

[48] Shacter, E. Quantification and significance of protein oxidation in biological samples. *Drug Metabolism Reviews,* 2000 32, 307–326.

[49] Lindhal, T. Endogenous damage to DNA. Philosophical Transactions of the Royal Society London, 1996 B351, 1529-1533.

[50] Stadtman, E R. Ascorbic acid and oxidative inactivation of proteins. *American Journal of Clinical Nutrition,* 1991 54, 1125S– 1128S.

[51] Peto, R; Doll, R; Buckley, JD; Sporn, MB. Can dietary beta-carotene materially reduce human cancer rates? *Nature.* 1981 290, 201.

[52] Block, G; Patterson, B; Subar, A. Fruit, vegetables and cancer prevention: a review of the epidemiological evidence. *Nutri. Cancer.* 1992 18, 1.

[53] Rice-Evans, CA; Miller, NJ; Paganga, G. Structure-antioxidant activity relationships of flavonoids and phenolic acids. *Free Radical Biology and Medicine,* 1996 20, 933.

[54] Mayne, ST. Beta-carotene, carotenoids, and disease prevention in humans. *FASEB Journal,* 1996 10, 690.

[55] Stocker, R. The ambivalence of vitamin E in atherogenesis. *TIBS,* 1999 24, 219.

[56] Pietta, PG. Flavonoids as antioxidants. *Journal of Natural Products,* 2000 63, 1035.

[57] Otero, P; Viana, M; Herrera, E; Bonet, B. Antioxidant and prooxidant effects of ascorbic acid, dehydroascorbic acid and flavonoids on LDL submitted to different degrees of oxidation. *Free Radical Research.* 1997 27, 619–626.

[58] Halliwell, B. The antioxidant paradox. *Lancet,* 2000 355, 1179-1180.

[59] Beatty, ER; England, TG; Geissler, CA; Aruoma, OI; Halliwell, B. Effects of antioxidant vitamin supplementation on markers of DNA damage and plasma antioxidants. *Proceedings of the Nutrition Society,* 1999 58, 44.

[60] Rehman, A; Collis, CS; Yang, M. The effects of iron and vitamin C co-supplementation on oxidative damage to DNA in healthy volunteers. *Biochemisty Biophysics Research Communications,* 1998 246, 293–98.

[61] Podmore, ID; Griffiths, HR; Herbert, KE; Mistry, N; Mistry, P; Lunec, J. Vitamin C exhibits pro-oxidant properties. *Nature,* 1998 392, 559.

[62] Prieme, H; Loft, S; Nyyssonen, K; Salonen, JT; Poulsen, HE. No effect of supplementation with vitamin E, ascorbic acid or coenzyme Q on oxidative DNA damage estimated by 8-oxo-7,8-dihydro-2-deoxyguanosine excretion in smokers. *American Journal of Clinical Nutrition,* 1997 65, 503–507.

[63] Steinbrecher, UP; Zhang, H; Lougheed, M. Role of oxidative modified LDL in atherosclerosis. *Free Radical Biology and Medicine.* 1990 9, 155-168.

[64] Esterbauer, H; Gebicki, J; Puhl, H; Jurgens, G. The role of lipid peroxidation and antioxidants in oxidative modification of LDL. *Free Radical Biology and Medicine.* 1992 13, 341–90.

[65] Frei, B. Vitamin C as an antiatherogen: mechanisms of action. In: Packer L; Fuchs J. editors. Vitamin C in health and disease. New York: Marcel Dekker Inc; 1997;163–82.

[66] Jialal, I; Vega, GL; Grundy, SM. Physiologic levels of ascorbate inhibit the oxidative modification of low density lipoprotein. *Atherosclerosis,* 1990 82, 185–191.

[67] Frei, B; Gaziano, JM. Content of antioxidants, preformed lipid hydroperoxides, and cholesterol as predictors of the susceptibility of human LDL to metal ion-dependent and -independent oxidation. *Journal of Lipid Research,* 1993 34, 2135–2145,

[68] Lehr, HA; Frei, B; Arfors, KE. Vitamin C prevents cigarette smoke-induced leukocyte aggregation and adhesion to endothelium in vivo. *Proceedings of the National Academy of Sciences U.S.A.,* 1994 91, 7688-7692.

[69] Lehr, HA; Weyrich, AS; Saetzler, RK; Jurek, A; Arfors, KE; Zimmerman, GA; Prescott, SM; McIntyre, TM. Vitamin C blocks inflammatory platelet-activating factor mimetics created by cigarette smoking. *The Journal of Clinical Investigation,* 1997 99, 2358-2364.

[70] Lehr, HA; Frei, B; Olofsson, AM; Carew, TE; Arfors, KE. Protection from oxidized LDL induced leukocyte adhesion to microvascular and macrovascular endothelium in vivo by vitamin C but not by vitamin E. *Circulation,* 1995 91, 1552-1532.

[71] Steinberg, D. Low density lipoprotein oxidation and its pathobiological significance. *Journal of Biological Chemistry,* 1997 272, 20963–20966.

[72] Steinberg, D; Lewis, A. Conner Memorial Lecture. Oxidative modification of LDL and atherogenesis. *Circulation,* 1997 95, 1062–1071.

[73] Chisolm, GM; Steinberg, D. The oxidative modification hypothesis of atherogenesis: an overview. *Free Radical Biology and Medicine,* 2000 28, 1815– 1826.

[74] Crawford, RS; Kirk, EA; Rosenfeld, ME; LeBoeuf, RC; Chait, A. Dietary antioxidants inhibit development of fatty streak lesions in the LDL receptor-deficient mouse. *Arteriosclerosis, Thrombosis, and Vascular Biology,* 1998 18, 1506–1513.

[75] Mahfouz, MM; Kawano, H; Kummerow, FA. Effect of cholesterol rich diets with and without added vitamins E and C on the severity of atherosclerosis in rabbits. *American Journal of Clinical Nutrition,* 1997 66, 1240–1249.

[76] Frei, B; England, L; Ames, BN. Ascorbate is an outstanding antioxidant in human blood plasma. *Proceedings of the National Academy of Sciences U.S.A.,* 1989 86, 6377-6381.

[77] Wayner, DD; Burton, GW; Ingold, KU; Barclay, LRC; Locke, SI. The relative contribution of vitamin E, urate, ascorbate, and proteins to the total peroxyl radical-trapping antioxidant activity of human blood plasma. *Biochimica et Biophysica Acta,* 1987 924, 408-19.

[78] Lambelet, P; Saucy, F; Lolliger, I. Chemical evidence for interactions between vitamin E and C. *Experentia,* 1985 41, 13384-13388.

[79] Darley-Usmar, V; Halliwell, B. Blood radicals. *Pharmacological Research,* 1996 13, 649-657.

[80] Maxwell SR. Coronary artery disease-free radical damage, antioxidant protection and the role of homocysteine. *Basic Research in Cardiology,* 2000 95 (Suppl 1), I65–I71.

[81] Brown, AA; Hu, FB. Dietary modulation of endothelial function: implications for cardiovascular disease. *American Journal of Clinical Nutrition,* 2001 73, 673-686.

[82] Drexler, H; Hornig, B. Endothelial dysfunction in human disease. *Journal of Molecular Cell Cardiology,* 1999 31, 51–60.

[83] Ness, A; Egger, M; Davey-Smith, G. Role of antioxidant vitamins in prevention of cardiovascular disease. *British Medical Journal,* 1999 319, 577-579.

[84] Marnett, LJ. Peroxy free radicals: Potential mediators of tumor initiation and promotion. *Carcinogenesis,* 1987 8, 1365–1373.

[85] Tappel, AL. Lipid peroxidation damage to cell components. *Fed. Proc.,* 1973 32, 1870–1874.

[86] Woodall, AA; Ames, BN. Diet and oxidative damage to DNA: the importance of ascorbate as an antioxidant. In: Packer, L; Fuchs, J. editors. *Vitamin C in health and disease.* New York: Marcel Dekker Inc; 1997; 193–203.

[87] IARC Handbooks of Cancer Prevention, volume 2, Carotenoids. Lyon, France: International Agency for Research on Cancer; 1998; 137–219.

[88] Niki, E. Antioxidants in the relation to lipid peroxidation. *Chemistry and Physics of Lipids,* 1987 44, 227–253.

[89] Cameron, E; Pauling, L. Ascorbic acid and the glycosaminoglycans. *Oncology,* 1973 27, 181-192.

[90] Block, G. Vitamin C and cancer prevention: the epidemiological evidence. *American Journal of Clinical Nutrition,* 1991 53, 270S-282S.

[91] Uddin, S, Ahmad, S. Antioxidant protection against cancer and other human diseases. *Comprehensive Therapy,* 1995 21, 41-45.

[92] Bendich, A. Vitamin C safety in humans. In: Packer, L; Fuchs, J, editors. *Vitamin C in health and disease.* New York: Marcel Dekker Inc; 1997; 367-79.

[93] Sobala, GM; Schorah, CJ; Shires, S; Lynch, DA; Gallacher, B; Dixon, MF; Axon, AT. Effect of eradication of Helicobacter pylori on gastric juice ascorbic acid concentrations. *Gut,* 1993 34, 1038–1041.

[94] Pannala, AS. Inhibition of ONOO- mediated tyrosine nitration by catechin polyphenols *Biochemical and Biophysical Research Communications.* 1997 232, 164- 172.

[95] Helser, MA; Hotchkiss, JH; Roe, DA. Influence of fruit and vegetable juices on the endogenous formation of N-nitrosoproline and N-nitrosothiazolidine-4-carboxylic acid in humans on controlled diets. *Carcinogenesis,* 1992 13, 2277–2280,

[96] Tsao, CS. Inhibiting effect of ascorbic acid on growth of human mammary tumor xenografts. *American Journal of Clinical Nutrition,* 1991 54, 1274S-1280S.

[97] Park, CH; Kimler, BF. Growth modulation of human leukemic, pre-leukemic and myeloma progenitor cell by L-ascorbic acid. *American Journal of Clinical Nutrition,* 1991 54, 1241S-1246S.

[98] Pavelic, K. L-ascorbic acid induced DNA strand breaks and cross links in human neuroblastoma cell. *Brain Research,* 1985 342, 369-373.

[99] Medina, MA; de Veas, RG; Schweigerer, L. Ascorbic acid is cytotoxic for peidoatric tumor cells cultured in vitro. *Biochemistry and Molecular Biology International,* 1994 34, 871-874.

[100] Liehr, JG. Vitamin C reduces the incidence and severity of renal tumors induced by estradiol or diethylstibesterol. *American Journal of Clinical Nutrition,* 1991 54, 1256S-1260S.

[101] McMichael, M; Moore, RM. Ischemia-reperfusion injury pathophysiology, Part I. *Journal of Veterinary Emergency Critical Care,* 2004 14, 231.

[102] Paller, MS; Hoidal, JR; Ferris, TF. Oxygen free radicals in ischemic acute renal failure in the rat. *Journal of Clinical Investigation,* 1984 74, 1156.

[103] Korkmaz, A; Kolankaya, D. The Protective Effects of Ascorbic Acid against Renal Ischemia-Reperfusion Injury in Male Rats. *Renal Failure,* 2009 31, 36-43.

[104] Halliwell, B. Drug Antioxidant effects. A basis for drug selection? *Drugs,* 1991 42, 569-581.

[105] Molyneux, CA; Glyn, MC; Ward, BJ. Oxidative stress and cardiac microvascular structure in ischemia/reperfusion: The protective effect of antioxidant vitamins. *Microvascular Research,* 2002 64, 265–277.

[106] Tata, V; Brizzi, S; Alessandra, L; Fierabracci, V; Malvaldi, G; Casini, A. Protective role of dehydroascorbate in rat liver ischemia/reperfusion injury. *Journal of Surgical Research,* 2005 123, 215–221.

[107] Huang, J; Agus, DB; Winfree, CJ; Kiss, S; Mack, WJ, McTaggart, RA; Choudhri, TF; Kim, LJ; Mocco, J; Pinsky, DJ; Fox, WD; Israel, RJ; Boyd, TA; Golde, DW; Connolly, ES Jr. Dehydroascorbic acid, a blood brain barrier transportable form of vitamin C, mediates potent cerebroprotection in experimental stroke. *Proceedings of the National Academy of Sciences U.S.A.,* 2001 98, 11720-11724.

[108] Clark, RAF. The molecular and cellular biology of wound repair. 2nd edition. New York: Plenum Press; 1996.

[109] Phillips, C; Pinnell, SR. Effects of ascorbic acid on proliferation and collagen synthesis in relation to the donor age of human dermal fibroblasts. *Society for Investigative Dermatology,* 1994 103, 228-232.

[110] Hellman, L; Burns, JJ. Metabolism of L-ascorbic acid-1-C14 in man. *Journal of Biological Chemistry,* 1958 230, 923-930.

[111] Taylor, A; Dorey, CK; Nowell, T. Oxidative stress and ascorbate in relation to risk for cataract and age-related maculopathy. In: Packer, L; Fuchs, J. editors. *Vitamin C in health and disease.* New York: Marcel Dekker Inc; 1997; 231–264.

[112] Taylor, A. Cataract: relationship between nutrition and oxidation. *Journal of American College Nutrition,* 1993 12,138-145.

[113] Spector, A. Oxidative stress induced cataract: mechanism of action. *FASEB Journal,* 1995 9, 1173-1178.

[114] Hankinson, SE; Stampfer, MJ; Seddon, JM. Nutrient intake and cataract extraction in women:a prospective study. *British Medical Journal,* 1992 305, 335–339.

[115] Robertson, JM, Donner, AP; Trevithick, JR. Vitamin E intake and risk of cataracts in humans. Annual New York Academy of Science

[116] Aruoma, OI. Pro-oxidant properties: an important consideration for food additives and/or nutrient components?. In Aruoma, OI; Halliwell B, editors. *Free Radicals and Food Additives.* London: Taylor and Francis; 1991, 173-194

[117] Halliwell, B; and Gutteridge, JMC. Free Radicals in Biology and Medicine. Oxford: Clarendon Press; 1989.

[118] Cooke, M S; Evans, MD; Podmore, ID; Herbert, KE; Mistry, N; Mistry, P; Hickenbotham, PT; Hussieni, A; Griffiths, HR ;Lunec, J. Novel repair action of vitamin C upon in vivo oxidative DNA damage. *FEBS Letters,* 1998, 439, 363– 367.

[119] Loft, S; Vistisen, K; Ewertz, M; Tjonneland, A; Overvad, K; Poulsen, HE. Oxidative DNA damage estimated by 8-hydroxydeoxyguanosine excretion in humans: influence of smoking, gender and body mass index. *Carcinogenesis,* 1992 13, 2241–2247.

[120] Halliwell B. How to characterize a biological antioxidant. *Free Radical Research Communications,* 1990, 9, 1-32.

[121] Colpo, E; de Bem, AF; Pieniz, S; Schettert, SD; dos Santos, RM; Farias, IL; Bertoncello, I; Moreira, CM; Barbosa, NV; Moretto, MB; Rocha, JB. A single high dose of ascorbic acid and iron is not correlated with oxidative stress in healthy volunteers. *Annual Nutrition Metabolism,* 2008 53(2), 79-85.

[122] Emerit, J; Beaumont, C; Trivin, F. Iron metabolism, free radicals, and oxidative injury. *Biochemical Pharmacology,* 2001 55, 333–339.

[123] Chen, K; Suh, J; Carr, AC; Marow, JD; Zeind, J; Frei, B. Vitamin C suppresses lipid damage in vivo even in the presence of iron over-load. *Americam Journal of Physiology- Endocrinology asn Metabolism,* 2000 279, 406-12.

[124] Johnson, RM; Goyette, G Jr, Ravindranath, Y; Ho, YS. Hemoglobin autoxidation and regulation of endogenous H 2 O 2 levels in erythrocytes. *Free Radical Biology and Medicine,* 2005 39, 1407–1417.

[125] Sinha, S; Saxena, R. Effect of iron on lipid peroxidation, and enzymatic and non-enzymatic antioxidants and bacoside-A content in medicinal plant Bacopa monnieri L. *Chemosphere,* 2006 62, 1340–1350.

[126] Samuni, A; Aronovitch, J; Godinger, D; Chevion, M; Czapski, G. On the cytotoxicity of vitamin C and metal ions. A site-specific Fenton mechanism. *European Journal of Biochemistry,* 1983 137, 119–124.

[127] Halliwell B. Free radicals and metal ions in health and disease. *Proceedings of the Nutrition Society,* 1987 46, 13-26.

[128] Higson, FK; Kohen, R; Chevion, M. Iron enhancement of ascorbate toxicity. *Free Radical Research Communication,* 198 5, 107-115.

[129] Rietjens, I; Boersma, M; de Haan, L; Spenkelink, B; Awad, H; Cnubbe, N; van Zanden, J; van der Woude, H; Alink, G; Koeman, J. The pro-oxidant chemistry of the natural antioxidants vitamin C, vitamin E,

carotenoids and flavonoids. *Environmental Toxicology and. Pharmacology,* 2002 11, 321-333.

[130] Nelson, SK; McCord, JM. Iron, oxygen radicals, and disease. *Advance Molecular Cell Biology,* 1998 25, 157–183.

[131] Niki, E. Action of ascorbic acid as a scavenger of active and stable oxygen radicals. *American Journal of Clinical Nutrition,* 1991 54 (suppl), 1119-1124.

[132] McCord, M. In: Iron free radicals, and oxidative injury. *Hematology,* 1998 35, 5–12.

[133] Gutteridge, JMC; Rowley, DA; Halliwell, B. Superoxide-dependent formation of hydroxyl radical and lipid peroxidation in the presence of iron salt: detection of catalytic iron and antioxidant activity in extracellular fluids. *Biochemical Journal,* 1982 206, 605–609.

[134] Herbert, V; Shaw, S; Jayatilleke, E. Vitamin C driven free radical generation from iron. *Journal of Nutrition,* 1996 126,1213-1220.

[135] Martin, A; Frei, B. Both intracellular and extracellular vitamin C inhibit atherogenic modification of LDL by humanvascular endothelial cells. *Arteriosclerosis, Thrombosis, and Vascular Biology,* 1997 17,1583-1590.

[136] Stait, SE; Leake, DE. Ascorbic acid can either increase or decrease low density lipoprotein modification. *FEBS Letters,* 1994 341, 263-267.

[137] Stich, HF; Wei, L; Whiting, RF. Enhancement of the chromosome-damaging action of ascorbate by transition metals. *Cancer Research,* 1979, 39, 4145-4151.

[138] Zhao, MJ; Jung, L. Kinetics of the competitive degradation of deoxyribose and other molecules by hydroxyl radicals produced by the fenton reaction in the presence of ascorbic acid. *Free Radical Research,* 1995 23, 229–243.

[139] Bijur, GN; Ariza, ME; Hitchcock, CL; Williams, MV. Antimutagenic and promutagenic activity of ascorbic acid during oxidative stress. *Environmental and Molecular Mutagenesis,* 1997 30, 339–345.

[140] Baysal, E; Sullivan, SG; Stern, A. Prooxidant and antioxidant effects of ascorbate on tert-butylhydroperoxideinduced erythrocyte membrane damage. *International Journal of Biochemistry.* 1989 21, 1109–1113.

[141] Laudicina, DC; Marnett, LJ. Enhancement of hydroperoxide-dependent lipid peroxidation in rat liver microsomes by ascorbic acid. *Archieves of Biochemistry and Biophyscics.* 1990 278, 73-80. 35.

[142] Yen, G; Duh, P; Tsai, H. Antioxidant and pro-oxidant properties of ascorbic acid and gallic acid, *Food Chemistry,* 2002 79, 307–313.

[143] Sahu, SC; Washington, MC. Iron-mediated oxidative DNA damage detected by fluorometric analysis of DNA unwinding in isolated rat liver nuclei. *Biomedical and Environmental Sciences,* 1991 4(3), 232-41.

[144] Zhang, P; Omaye, ST; β-Carotene: interactions with α-tocopherol and ascorbic acid in microsomal lipid peroxidation. *Journal of Nutritional Biochemistry,* 2001 12, 38–45.

[145] Sakagami, H; Satoh, K; Fukuchi, K; Gomi, K; Takeda, M. Effect of an iron chelator on ascorbate induced cytotoxicity, *Free Radical Biology and Medicine,* 1997 23, 260–270.

[146] Akatov, VS; Medvedev, AI; Solov'eva, ME; Merkushina, AI; Leshchenko, VV. Apoptotic death of human lympholeukemia HL-60 cells resultant from combined effect of cobalt octa-4,5-carboxyphthalocyanine propylenglycol ether and ascorbate. *Bulletin of Experimental Biology and Medicine,* 2005 140, 729-732.

[147] De Laurenzi, V; Melino, G; Savini, Y; Annicchiarico-Petruzzelli, M; Finazzi-Agrò, A; Avigliano, L. Cell death by oxidative stress and ascorbic acid regeneration in human neuroectodermal cell lines. *European Journal of Cancer,* 1995 4, 463–466.

[148] Lefebvre, Y; Pezerat, H. Production of activated species of oxygen during the chromate(VI)-ascorbate reaction: implication in carcinogenesis. *Chemical Research in Toxicology,* 1992 5,461-463.

[149] Park, SW; Lee, SM. Antioxidant and prooxidant properties of ascorbic acid on hepatic dysfunction induced by cold ischemia/reperfusion. *European Journal of Pharmacology,* 2008 580, 401-406.

[150] Gipp, WF; Pond, WG; Kallfelz, FA. Effect of dietary copper, iron, and ascorbic acid levels on hematology, blood, tissue copper, iron, and zinc concentrations and 64Cu and 59Fe metabolism in young pigs. *Journal of Nutrition,* 1974 104, 532–541.

[151] Suzuki, T; Yoshida, A. Effectiveness of dietary iron and ascorbic acid in the prevention and cure of moderately long-term toxicity in rats. *Journal of Nutrition,* 1979 109, 1974–1979.

[152] Erdogan, Z; Erdogan, S; Celik, S; Unlu, A. Effects of ascorbic Acid on cadmium-induced oxidative stress and performance of broilers. *Biological Trace Element Research,* 2005 104(1), 19–32.

[153] Kang, SA; Jang, YJ; Park, H. In vitro dual effects of Vitamin C on paraquat- induced lung damage: dependence on released metals from the damaged tissue. *Free Radical Research,* 1998 28, 93–107.

[154] Takahashi, O. Haemorrhagic toxicity of a large dose ofα-, β-,γ- and δ-tocopherols, ubiquinone, β-carotene, retinol acetate and L-ascorbic acid in the rat. *Food and Chemical Toxicology,* 1995 33,121–128.

[155] Premkumar, K; Bowlus, CL. Ascorbic acid reduces the frequency of iron induced micronuclei in bone marrow cells of mice. *Mutation Research,* 2003 542, 99–103.

[156] Chatterjee, GC; Chatterjee, S; Chatterjee, K; Sahu, A. Studies on the protective effects of ascorbic acid in rubidium toxicity. Toxicology and Applied Pharmacology, 1979 51, 47–58.

[157] Elhaïmeur, F; Courdet-Masuyer, C; Nicod, L; Guyon, C; Richert, L; Berthelot, A. Dietary vitamin C supplementation decreases blood pressure in DOCA-salt hypertensive male Sprague-Dawley rats and this is associated with increased liver oxidative stress. *Molecular Cell Biochemistry,* 2002 237, 77–83.

[158] Nowak, D; Pietras, T; Antczak, A; Piasecka, G; Król, M. Ascorbic acid did not alter the content of conjugated dienes and malondialdehyde in organs of mice. *Polish Journal of Pharmacology and Pharmacy,* 1992 44(5), 539-42.

[159] Young, IS; Torney, JJ; Trimble, ER. The effect of ascorbate supplementation on oxidative stress in the streptozotocin diabetic rat. *Free Radical Biology and Medicine,* 1992 13, 41-46.

[160] Speit, G; Wolf, M; Vogel, W. The sce-inducing capacity of vitamin C: Investigations in vitro and in vivo. *Mutation Research,* 1980 78:273.

[161] Galloway, SM; Painter RB. The use of short-term tests to measure the preventive action of reducing agents on formation and activation of carcinogenic nitroso compounds. *Mutation Research,* 1979 57, 57–67.

[162] Atkinson, A; Roy, D. In vivo DNA adducts formation by bisphenol A. *Environmental and Molecular Mutagenesis,* 1995 26, 60–66.

[163] Hasselberg, L; Meier, S; Svardal, A. Effects of alkylphenols on redox status in first spawning Atlantic cod (Gadus morhua). *Aquatic Toxicolgy,* 2004 69, 95–105.

[164] Aydoğan, M; Korkmaz, A; Barlas, N; Kolankaya, D. Pro-oxidant effect of vitamin C coadministration with bisphenol A, nonylphenol, and octylphenol on the reproductive tract of male rats. *Drug and Chemical Toxicology* (in press), DOI 10.3109/01480540903286468, 2010 .

[165] Appenroth, D; Winnefeld, K; Schroter, H; Rost, M. The ambiguous effect of ascorbic acid on chromate induced proteinuria in rats. *Archieves of Toxicology,* 1994 68, 138–141.

[166] Song, JH; Shin, SH; Ross, GM. Prooxidant effects of ascorbate in rat brain slices, *Journal of Neuroscience Research,* 1999 58, 328–336.

[167] Aydoğan, M; Korkmaz, A; Barlas, N; Kolankaya, D. The effect of vitamin C on bisphenol A, nonylphenol and octylphenol induced brain damages of male rats. *Toxicology,* 2008 249, 35–39.

[168] Korkmaz, A; Aydoğan, M; D. Kolankaya, D; Barlas, N. Vitamin C co-administration augments bisphenol A, nonylphenol and octylphenol induced oxidative damage on kidney of rats. *Environmental Toxicology.* (in pres) DOI: 10.1002/tox.20556, 2010.

[169] Cooke, MS; Mistry, N; Ahmad, J; Waller, H; Langford, L; Bevan, RJ;Evans, MD; Jones, GD; Herbert, KE; Griffiths, HR; Lunec, J. Deoxycytidine glyoxal: lesion induction and evidence of repair following vitamin C supplementation in vivo, *Free Radical Biology and Medicine,* 2003 34, 218–225.

[170] Childs, A; Jacobs, C; Kaminski, T; Halliwell B; Leeuwenburgh, C. Supplementation with vitamin C and N-acetyl-cysteine increases oxidative stress in humans after an acute muscle injury induced by eccentric exercise, *Free Radical Biology and Medicine,* 2001 31, 745–753

[171] Lamas GA; Ackermann, A. Clinical evaluation of chelation therapy: is there any wheat amidst the chaff?, *American Heart Journal,* 2000 140, 4–5.

[172] Rozema, TC. The protocol for safe and effective administration of EDTA and other chelating agents for vascular disease, degenerative disease and metal toxicity, *Journal of Advanced Medicine,* 1997 10, 11–17.

[173] Sardi, B. High-dose vitamin C and iron overload, *Annals of Internal Medicine,* 2004 140, 846–847.

[174] Naidu, KA. Vitamin C in human health and disease is still a mystery ? An overview, *Nutrition Journal,* 2003 2, 7.

[175] Hininger, I; Chollat-Namy, A; Sauvaigo, S; Osman, M; Faure, H; Cadet, J; Favier A; Roussel, AM. Assessment of DNA damage by comet assay on frozen total blood: method and evaluation in smokers and non-smokers, *Mutation Research,* 2004 558, 75–80.

[176] Chen, WT; Lin, YF; Yu, FC; Kao, WY; Huang WH; Yan, HC. Effect of ascorbic acid administration in hemodialysis patients on in vitro oxidative stress parameters: influence of serum ferritin levels, *American Journal of Kidney Diseases,* 2003 42, 158–166.

[177] Lachili, B; Hininger, I; Faure, H; Arnaud, J; Richard, MJ; Favier, A; Roussel, AM. Increased lipid peroxidation in pregnant women after iron and vitamin C supplementation, Biological Trace. *Element Research,* 2001 83, 103–110.

Index

S

T

Contents

KT-913-145

90 0498014 X

Language-learning

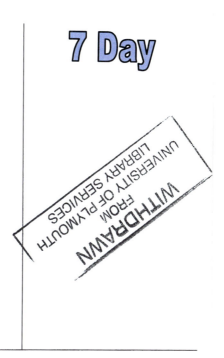

7 Day

University of Plymouth Library

Subject to status this item may be renewed
via your Voyager account

http://voyager.plymouth.ac.uk

Exeter tel: (01392) 475049
Exmouth tel: (01395) 255331
Plymouth tel: (01752) 232323

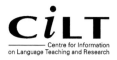
Centre for Information
on Language Teaching and Research

The Centre for Information on Language Teaching and Research (CILT)
provides a complete range of services for language professionals in every stage
and sector of education, and in business, in support of its brief to promote
Britain's foreign language capability.

CILT is a registered charity, supported by Central Government grants. CILT is
based in Covent Garden, London, and its services are delivered through a
national collaborative network of regional Comenius Centres in England, the
National Comenius Centre of Wales, Scottish CILT and Northern Ireland
CILT.

SCHML
Standing Conference of
Heads of Modern Languages
in Universities

SCHML (the Standing Conference of Heads of Modern Languages in
Universities) is an established professional association. Its activities are focused
on leadership and management issues of interest to all language providers in
the higher education sector (language departments and language centres).
Working in close collaboration with UCML (the University Council of
Modern Languages) and the new Subject Centre for Language, Linguistics
and Area Studies, SCHML aims to provide a support network and interactive
staff development for all those involved in the management of languages in
higher education.

CILT Publications are available through all good booksellers or directly from:

Central Books, 99 Wallis Rd,
London E9 5LN.
Tel: 020 8986 4854. Fax: 020 8533 5821.

LANGUAGE-
LEARNING
FUTURES

Issues and strategies for modern languages provision in higher education

Edited by   James A Coleman
Derrik Ferney
David Head
Rob Rix

C*i*LT
Centre for Information
on Language Teaching and Research

SCHML
Standing Conference of
Heads of Modern Languages
in Universities

First published in 2001 by the Centre for Information on Language Teaching and Research, 20 Bedfordbury, London WC2N 4LB in association with the Standing Conference of Heads of Modern Languages in Universities (SCHML).

ISBN 1 902031 87 3

2005 2004 2003 2002 / 10 9 8 7 6 5 4 3 2 1

Printed in Great Britain by Copyprint (UK) Ltd.

CILT Publications are available from: **Central Books**, 99 Wallis Rd, London E9 5LN. Tel: 020 8986 4854. Fax: 020 8533 5821. Book trade representation (UK and Ireland): **Broadcast Book Services**, Charter House, 27a London Road, Croydon CR0 2RE. Tel: 020 8681 8949. Fax: 020 8688 0615.

Introduction: university language teaching and learning in the twentieth and twenty-first centuries

James A Coleman and David Head

When the mileometer in their car clicks round to a number ending in several zeros, some drivers reflect for a moment on the distance travelled and places visited, before looking ahead to likely future routes. So with the year 2000: whether or not it has any real significance, it has provided many people, university linguists amongst them, with an opportunity to reflect on past developments and future directions.

One hundred years ago, the study of modern languages was virtually unknown in British universities. The discipline was introduced cautiously, against opposition, and could only be made acceptable by adopting the precise teaching pattern of classical languages. Its inferiority was marked by the label 'modern', which became so firmly attached that it still lingers, although the classical disciplines have now shrunk to marginal significance in the overall scheme of university study. The curriculum embraced philology, the historical canon of 'great' texts, and language learning based on paradigmatic grammar, on drills and on two-way translation.

The model proved durable, even as institutions which for decades had delivered external London degrees became universities in their own right. When the present editors were themselves students, virtually all language degrees had an exclusively literary focus. In the mid 1960s, when barely one in twenty of the age cohort attended university, combined honours courses were few and far between and regarded as an option for the weaker students. The grammar-translation method dominated the language classroom, oral-aural skills were a matter of 'conversation classes' and a year's assistantship was an interlude during which twentieth-century students were deemed to pick up spoken language as their predecessors had picked up Canalettos and an insight into sex. Ever the exception, Oxford and Cambridge tested oral skills only on entry and actively discouraged students from diluting their academic studies by going abroad.

2 LANGUAGE-LEARNING FUTURES

The standard French coursebook, Niklaus and Wood's *French prose composition*, comprised 158 English texts for translation into French. Although divided into 'Narrative', 'Critical', 'Philosophical', etc, and despite a few examples of journalism from the *Times* and the *Manchester Guardian*, the texts shared a predominantly literary style: the 'Conversational' section consisted exclusively of literary dialogue. The 1966 reprint was entirely unchanged from the original 1936 publication and the preface asserted: 'We have not included a vocabulary, or notes or hints of any kind, because they tend to promote stereotyped translation rather than to encourage original thought'. For grammar, students turned to Mansion's *A grammar of present day French*, first published in 1916.

The pace of change in language teaching has accelerated since then. The first revolution in syllabuses came in the late 1960s, and not from the UK's then 'new' universities, but from the new polytechnics and the colleges of advanced technology which had just won university status. Instead of a purely literary diet, students could opt for Area Studies, or Applied Language Studies, with a practical, career-oriented outcome. Overall student numbers expanded slowly through the 1970s and 1980s, although, following expansion in the 1960s, a near-freeze applied to staff appointments from the mid-1970s until the mid-1990s. Curricula became more varied, with a language more often linked to another language or a professional discipline. The language laboratories of the 1960s were supplemented by satellite television and video in the 1980s, and by widespread use of Computer-Assisted Language Learning by the end of the 1980s. At about the same time, the language departments in Polytechnics and colleges, under the banner of their Standing Conference of Heads of Modern Languages (SCHML), introduced language programmes for specialists in other disciplines, which became known as Institution-Wide Languages Programmes (IWLPs). By 1992, the year in which British polytechnics gained university status, there were more non-specialists than specialist linguists (Thomas, 1993).

The early 1990s saw the Open University finally introduce language courses and a huge expansion in student numbers in what were by now ex-polytechnics. Curricula nationally were modularised and semesterised and independent learning became more central on resource grounds if not for academic reasons. Throughout the decade (Coleman, 1996), single honours courses diminished in favour of joint, combined or modular courses. The introduction of a National Curriculum in schools, with a foreign language among the core subjects, replaced to some extent the elitism which had previously reserved language study for the most fortunate, but failed to deliver the numbers of eager language students for whom universities had expanded to make room. Recruitment to specialist language courses peaked in 1992 and the slow decline which followed, at least for French, German and Russian, became a steep decline in 1999 and 2000. At the start of the new millennium, as the report of the Nuffield Languages Inquiry (Nuffield Foundation, 2000) has shown, languages in UK higher education were in crisis. The increasing mismatch in staffing between the demand for applied linguists and the supply of literary PhDs, documented by Michael Kelly for the University Council of Modern Languages (itself created in 1993 as an over-arching body of departments and professional associations to lobby for higher education languages in all domains) has become all but irrelevant as no new posts are created. Furthermore, few replacements are allowed for the retiring 1960s intake of staff, and closures and redundancies reduce the universities' ability to deliver the specialist and non-specialist linguists which, as the Nuffield survey shows, the United Kingdom badly needs.

Meanwhile external assessment had come to both teaching and research. The Research Assessment Exercises which now dominate the lives of most UK academics began in 1986. The fifth takes place in 2001, with research into language pedagogy assured of a respectable consideration for the first time. The Quality Assessment process for teaching and learning, which saw most departments visited by a team of specialist assessors in 1995/96, has not yet become such an established feature of academic life, with revised arrangements to be implemented in 2003–6 still a matter of heated discussion. The creation of the Quality Assurance Agency for Higher Education from a forced marriage of its two rival predecessors ensured that new quality procedures would not be straightforward. The revisions of the specification for Benchmarking are an instance of the uncertainties which have marked the opening of the twenty-first century, although Benchmarking guidelines for languages will be produced shortly.

The creation of the Institute for Learning and Teaching in Higher Education should have marked increased professional recognition for teaching as against research: perhaps that is why it has met such fierce opposition in many traditional universities. Certainly, the position of research into language learning and teaching is little if any better than in the previous decades, with no funding body recognising applied linguistic research as its central concern.

On the teaching side, new initiatives brought more positive results. In 1997, the UK Funding Councils adopted ten language projects under the Fund for the Development of Teaching and Learning (FDTL), and charged them with spreading good practice and addressing problem areas. It was the FDTL projects which first proposed a conference in the year 2000 that would allow university linguists to take stock, look back and look ahead.

This volume has its origin in that ground-breaking international conference 'The New Communicators: Graduates with Languages. Teaching Modern Languages in Universities in the 21st century', which took place at the University of Nottingham, UK, in July 2000. The conference was sponsored not only by FDTL but also by

SCHML, UCML and the Centre for Information on Language Teaching and Research (CILT) – in other words by the principal bodies and agencies involved in university language teaching.

The summer 2000 conference was the opportunity not only to discuss the achievements of these projects, but also to expand the debate in order to encompass research on other crucial questions, ranging from autonomy, intercultural skills and distance learning to grammar teaching and learner motivation.

The chapters in the present volume are not published proceedings, but rather the development of some of the main ideas presented at the conference. As well as an evaluation of the FDTL languages programme, they provide an informed and up-to-date research perspective on a number of areas and offer fresh analyses of issues that are of central importance to the future of language teaching and learning in higher education.

In the first chapter, Jim Coleman reviews the work of the FDTL languages projects in the UK from 1997–2000. Representing the biggest single investment ever in modern languages within the UK, the projects sought to spread good practices and address problems in areas as diverse as residence abroad, independent learning, staff development, assessment and transferable skills for non-specialist language learners. Coleman evaluates the outcomes of the projects, both finite and longer term, shows how the projects sought to identify and promote best practice in their respective domains and reviews the obstacles to successful dissemination and the strategies which work best to achieve it.

Mark Bannister considers some of the ways in which the learning outcomes of the period of residence abroad can be better integrated into the overall course of study. He emphasises the centrality of autonomous learning as a means of improving linguistic competence and intercultural understanding during this key phase for the undergraduate language learner.

The label 'independent language learning' has for some time been used to refer to learning that is undertaken without any direct control by the teacher. David Little contends that this is very much an overstatement, for independent language learning will always require some form of social interaction and appropriate support from highly skilled teaching staff, and not just from technology, if it is to be effective.

Drawing on a national survey undertaken among staff in language departments in UK universities between Easter 1999 and Easter 2000, Nicole McBride investigates current practices in the language used in the teaching of 'content' or 'cultural' modules. In particular, she seeks to establish whether universities can address the challenge of producing language graduates who are able to operate effectively in other languages and cultures if they do not, as undergraduates, make regular use of the target language as a supporting feature of their studies.

Vicky Davies and Michael Jones discuss their experience of introducing the European Language Portfolio (ELP), an innovation which was called into being by the Committee of Ministers of the Council of Europe in 1998. The aim of the ELP was to create a means by which all learners would record their qualifications and 'other significant linguistic and cultural experiences' in an internationally transparent manner. Davies and Jones conclude that the ELP in addition equips students with an effective range of strategies which they are able to adapt to any given learning situation.

Marina Orsini-Jones and Glynis Cousin present the outcomes of a two-year investigation into language students' perception of their learning and discuss the implications for the creation of a powerful learning environment. They show that the key to achieving this is a collaborative approach that involves consulting students about their learning and then about the kind of teaching and interpersonal relationships they require in order to be able to learn effectively.

John Morley and Sandra Truscott report on a project which has set out to assess the quantity and quality of peer-generated corrective feedback in tandem language learning. They also present a set of guidelines for giving corrective feedback that can be used with students who are working on this type of collaborative learning scheme.

Taking her data from tandem learner diaries, Lesley Walker shows that language learning can be seen to flourish where there is a proactive partnership between peers and where effective learner strategies are in evidence. She concludes that tandem learning has moved learning methodology forward for the new millennium.

In the majority of UK universities which offer the study of Russian to degree level, students are admitted *ab initio* or with an advanced level of study in the language. They all initially follow a programme that is streamed for at least one year. Sarah Hudspith examines findings which suggest that *ab initio* students outperform their more experienced fellow students and also that the students who start from an advanced level have the greatest difficulties during the early streaming stages.

The subject of Nicola Reimann's contribution is the process of studying a language in the context of a university's Institution-Wide Languages Programme. She seeks to describe and understand whether there are any significant differences between university students who discontinue the study of German and those who continue from one year to another. The study seeks to ascertain the reasons for continuation and non-continuation. One of her main conclusions is that maximum continuation can only be achieved if students see language learning as a relevant and integral part of their education and are aware of the relevance of their language skills.

Inma Álvarez and Cecilia Garrido analyse ways of exposing language students to cultural issues with a view to enabling them to cross cultures confidently, using as their test-bed the development of a language programme that gives equal importance to linguistic and cultural content.

It is hoped that this collection will contribute to continued discussion of central issues in university language teaching and learning and sow seeds of ideas which will grow into papers for the next international conference, scheduled for 2002.

James A Coleman
David Head
February 2001

References

Coleman, J. A. (1996) *Studying languages: a survey. The proficiency, background, attitudes and motivations of students of foreign languages in the United Kingdom and Europe.* London: Centre for Information on Language Teaching and Research.

Thomas, G. (1993) *Survey of European languages in the United Kingdom 1992.* London: Council for National Academic Awards.

Lessons for the future: evaluating FDTL languages

James A Coleman ● *University of Portsmouth*

> *Well-established university teachers are the most difficult group for whom to provide suitable programmes of continuing staff development. Not only may cynicism have set in, but they will also be a very diverse group with very different sets of experience and expressed priorities.* (McKeachie, 1997 in Bradbeer, 1999: 19)

The Fund for the Development of Teaching and Learning (FDTL), established by the UK's Higher Education Funding Council for England (HEFCE), represents the biggest single investment ever in university modern languages, totalling around £2.25 million. This paper draws on the experience of all the FDTL language projects to answer the question: what have we done with the money? More specifically: what activities have FDTL language projects undertaken and what has been their impact?

In 1995/96, British university departments teaching modern foreign languages were visited as part of the university funding councils' Quality Assessment (QA) process (now renamed 'subject review'). Teams of trained language academics sought to evaluate the student learning experience through observation, documentation and discussion, awarding a grade from one (unacceptable) to four (excellent) on each of six 'Aspects of Provision': Curriculum Design, Content and Organisation; Teaching, Learning and Assessment; Student Progression and Achievement; Student Support and Guidance; Learning Resources; Quality Assurance and Enhancement. In England and Northern Ireland (Scotland and Wales adopted different procedures), 110 single-subject visits were carried out, while some institutions preferred to have all their modern language provision assessed at the same time (see Figure 1).

Subject	Single subject visits	Modern languages visits
French	30	45
German and related languages	30	45
Iberian languages and studies	21	38
Italian	15	19
Russian and Eastern European languages	14	15

Figure 1: Quality Assessment visits in modern languages, 1995/96

The process was imperfect, but each visit led to a published report and the conclusions of the individual reports were brought together in overview reports for each language, discussing the quality of the students' learning experience, identifying good practice and indicating where improvements might be made.

The FDTL sought to build on the QA process (though formally restricted, like QA, to England and Northern Ireland). In autumn 1997, after two rounds of open competition, ten projects in modern languages were allocated three-year government funding totalling over £2 million in order to spread the good practice identified in the QA process and to address those quality-assurance issues which the QA process had unearthed in such areas as residence abroad, integration of Information and Communication Technology (ICT) and independent learning or training of language assistants.

At each stage of the competition, co-operation between institutions was encouraged, but when the bids were evaluated in summer 1997, the sole criterion applied by the HEFCE was bid quality, not need. On the one hand, this meant there was a danger of duplication and overlap: and indeed, three projects were approved in each of the areas of residence abroad and independent learning. On the other hand, judging exclusively on the basis of bids' quality meant that some problems raised by the QA process might not be addressed: content teaching in the target language and the integration of language with content, for example, had been flagged up as requiring attention, but no projects in these areas were selected for funding. Perhaps more damaging to the whole exercise was the fact that area/cultural/literary/media studies – in other words all the activities undertaken by language departments beyond the teaching of the target language itself – would receive no funding and no attention under FDTL.

To exclude a major part of any academic discipline from a major national initiative is regrettable; that this should have happened with modern languages is particularly unfortunate, given the uniqueness of the subject. For unlike students in other disciplines, language graduates have not only acquired new skills and knowledge, but actually engaged their personal identity in their learning. The study of other subjects takes place within the home culture and in English: only languages take students into another culture, with classes in a foreign language. In no other university discipline are individual motivation and attitudes or social learning so important. And perhaps in no other discipline are there such significant divisions within the subject community.

Those who teach the language itself in UK universities are more likely to have a teaching qualification, and a professional and occasionally a research interest in teaching, than those who teach the 'content' element of modern-language degrees. They are also more likely to be without a research degree, to be on a part-time and/or fixed-term contract and to be teaching a large number of hours. 'Content' teachers will, in a majority of cases, have no teaching qualification, but hold a research degree and a research interest in some aspect of the literature, culture, media or sociology of the target-language culture. Language classes may figure within their lower teaching load, but many are indifferent to, or indeed scornful of, language teaching and learning, regarding it as the mechanical aspect of the discipline, one which makes few intellectual demands and is predominantly accomplished outside the classroom during students' residence abroad. This particular split, exemplified in the largest university language discipline, French, by the existence of three parallel subject associations researching the language, literature and society of Francophone cultures, has been deepened by the growing influence of the Research Assessment Exercise. First introduced in 1986 to scepticism and derision, it has since become the most significant element in the lives of most UK academics. With around £900 million per annum resting on the grades allocated to a department, it is small wonder that many departments have reduced teaching hours to allow 'content' staff to devote time to research outputs, typically putting more pressure on language-teaching staff.

Ironically, another unique feature of languages as a university discipline is the research effort which has gone into the study of language teaching and learning. A Boolean search of any university library catalogue combining a subject discipline 'x' with 'learning' or 'teaching' will produce, where x = language, a total greater than the combined total of all other disciplines taken together. Language teaching is a specialism in a sense which applies to the teaching of no other university subject.

In the context of this pre-existing division within university modern languages, memorably described as separate tribes in Evans's *Language people* (1988), an opportunity to build bridges by addressing teaching and learning issues outside the language domain seems to have been missed. All the FDTL language projects selected related either to generic issues such as staff development or specifically to language teaching and, especially when combined with the emphasis on innovation which the bidding process encouraged, could only make it harder for the FDTL programme to make an impact across the whole sector. How were projects to engage with traditional content and with the traditional methods for delivering content teaching? How were those in receipt of FDTL funding, many of them already specialists in teaching and learning, to involve a community whose principal activity was research and for whom intellectual energy, time, professional status and indeed a great deal of institutional income attached to research and not to improving the learning experience? Since their research topics and their teaching topics were not covered by the FDTL programme, who could blame them if they chose to ignore it? The danger was, then, from the very start, that HEFCE's selection procedure would itself leave successful bidders preaching to the converted, ignored by the majority of those teaching within the discipline, with the existing barriers between language and 'content', between teaching and research largely intact, if not actually reinforced.

A further question must be how effective was the 'project' approach itself, with each successful bidder funded for a maximum of three years. Even if appropriately qualified staff can be recruited or seconded without delay, their commitment to a short-term project will be reduced. Some projects have had a high and disruptive turnover of staff seeking more secure long-term employment. Even those, such as the Residence Abroad Project, which have been fortunate enough to retain staff for a full three years, have seen colleagues who have built up unequalled subject expertise lost to the sector with the end of project funding.

A three-year cycle in itself creates problems of timing, particularly where residence abroad is concerned. In other circumstances, one might wish to identify good practices, evaluate them with a pilot group and analyse and disseminate the resulting recommendations. But in order to learn lessons from a pilot group of students who have followed an innovative programme integrating residence abroad, they had to be returning from the target country in October 1999, therefore abroad during the academic year 1998/99, which would have left only the first semester 1997/98 to identify good practices and build a learning programme incorporating them, so that the pilot group could follow the new programme of preparation in the second semester – an impossible schedule.

If the HEFCE FDTL programme suffered from built-in limitations on its own effectiveness, it also had a support mechanism: the National Co-ordination Team (NCT). With an initial brief relating to FDTL later extended to another initiative, the third phase of the Teaching and Learning Technology Programme (TLTP3), the NCT's dual role was to both support and monitor projects, and ultimately to help translate project-level activity into national policy. All projects benefited from briefings, discussion and advice through individual visits and telephone/e-mail contact and an annual conference which became far better focused and more useful during the three years of the projects' existence.

The ten projects have addressed five themes: residence abroad (3), independent learning (3), staff development (2), assessment and transferable skills for non-specialist language learners. The ALLADIN project, funded under TLTP3, joined the group from 1998. Individual projects were as follows in Figure 2.

Domain	Project name	Co-ordinating university	Website
Residence abroad	Interculture	Lancaster	www.lancs.ac.uk/ users/interculture/
Residence abroad	Learning and Residence Abroad (LARA)	Oxford Brookes	lara.fdtl.ac.uk/ lara/index.htm
Residence abroad	Residence Abroad Project (RAPPORT)	Portsmouth	www.hum.port.ac. uk/slas/rapport/
Independent learning	Curriculum and Independence for the Learner Support Network (CIEL)	Southampton	ciel.lang.soton.ac.uk
Independent learning	Strategies for Managing an Independent Learning Environment (SMILE)	Hull	www.hull.ac.uk/ langinst/smile/index. htm
Independent learning	Web-Enhanced Language Learning (WELL)	Liverpool John Moores	www.well.ac.uk
Independent learning	Autonomous Language Learning in Art and Design Using Interactive Networks (ALLADIN)	Surrey Institute of Art and Design	www.surrart.ac.uk/ alladin
Staff development	Developing Excellence in Language Teaching through the Observation of Peers (DEVELOP)	Leeds Metropolitan	www.lmu.ac.uk/cls/ fdtl/develop/

Staff development	Development of Postgraduate and Language Assistants (DOPLA)	Birmingham	www.bham.ac.uk/ dopla
Assessment	Effective practices in assessment in modern languages: a German language perspective	Ulster	
Transferable skills for non-specialist language learners	Transferable Skills Development for Non-specialist Learners of Modern Languages (TransLang)	Central Lancashire	www.uclan.ac.uk/ facs/class/languages/ translang/tlweb.htm

The three residence abroad projects undertook joint activities under the nicely ambiguous title Residence Abroad Matters (http://ram.fdtl.ac.uk/).

Figure 2: FDTL projects in modern languages

Unfortunately, the context in which the projects began working was unfavourable in other respects too. The decline in numbers of students opting for a university degree course in modern languages, which was already beginning to become evident in 1997, had by 2000 become the worst crisis in the century or so of existence of modern languages as a university discipline. The reasons are diverse:

• a generally Eurosceptic and at times xenophobic climate created and maintained by several national newspapers, which contrasts strongly with the pro-European sentiments which accompanied the completion of the single market in 1992 and saw the highest ever levels of interest in foreign language study;

• the introduction of a foreign language into the core of the National Curriculum for secondary schools – although this might have been expected to enhance foreign language study, its indirect effect, in the view of many, was:

  – to contribute to a cramped timetable in which studying a second modern foreign language became all but impossible, so that fewer pupils (especially in the public sector) see themselves as potential language specialists;

  – to make it necessary to target the 16-plus GCSE exams at less-able pupils, and thus create a huge gap in level between GCSE and the 18-plus A level exams;

– to give pupils the impression that languages are a 'difficult' subject and that achieving a good A level is much harder than in other subjects – a perception borne out by statistics;

- the introduction of more appealing new subjects at A level, some of them perceived to be more interesting, easier and better related to the world of work;

- the inaccurate but widespread impression in schools that a language degree can lead only to a career in teaching or translating/interpreting – with the introduction of tuition fees, the replacement of grants with repayable loans and a general opinion that graduation is accompanied by substantial debt, future students and their parents or other financial backers are increasingly focusing on the employment opportunities which courses offer;

- the absence of role models competent in foreign languages:

  – sports and media personalities, whatever their nationality, are always interviewed in English;

  – a single, well-publicised speech in French by the Prime Minister in 1997 was followed by years in which no British statesman was ever shown using a foreign language;

  – whereas in schools elsewhere in Europe and in the wider world, teachers of other subjects typically speak additional languages, and in many places provide teaching through the medium of a second or foreign language, few teachers in British schools offer a language other than English, with the consequence that competence in a foreign language, widely perceived by pupils elsewhere as a transferable life skill alongside such skills as communication, problem solving or team working, is here seen as a school subject, and a particularly difficult one, offered by teachers many of whom are foreigners themselves.

Whatever their relative significance and whether or not traditionalism in university departments contributed, as was suggested as early as 1992 ('the nationwide boom in demand for language studies of all kinds is continuing to mask any student disenchantment with a predominantly literary syllabus', Coleman and Parker, 1992: 10), the combined impact of these factors has been to accelerate the trend away from single and joint/combined honours language degrees, a trend quantified by a major national study in the mid-1990s (Coleman, 1996: 35–36) and by evidence submitted to the Nuffield Languages Inquiry in 1998 (Towell, 1998). The final report of the Inquiry states bleakly that 'University language departments are closing, leaving the sector in deep crisis' (The Nuffield Languages Inquiry, 2000: 7).

A further contextual factor needs to be mentioned: the imbalance in funding and prestige between teaching and research. The majority of recurrent funding to universities is earmarked for teaching, but is released by an easily attained quality threshold. To enhance teaching and learning, some £30 million per annum is available, divided among institutional, individual and discipline-based initiatives, substantially dependent on competitive bidding and closely tied to pre-established budgets and activities. For research, on the other hand, some £900 million per annum is available and is distributed on a competitive basis with little restriction on how individual institutions choose to spend it. Small wonder that individual academics, their departments and universities mostly channel their efforts in a direction to which resources and prestige attach in greater quantity. In this sense, the funding councils themselves might be said to be undermining the impact of the FDTL programme: FDTL languages have encountered resistance in some places, have found senior academics unavailable because of research sabbaticals timed to help achieve results in the 2001 Research Assessment Exercise and, in a few cases, have actually met individuals who have been instructed not to work with FDTL but to devote time to research outputs instead.

Despite these two major inhibiting factors, FDTL Languages have succeeded in the task of identifying, evaluating, disseminating and promoting good practices. The plural *practices* has been adopted by all in recognition that there is no single ideal model, but rather a range of solutions, among which each institutional context determines those which are best suited. Dissemination, as the mixed record of earlier initiatives in higher education has confirmed, is not the final step of a programme: excellent products and approaches will not be taken up unless the potential user community is involved in their development from the start (the 'not invented here' syndrome). The need to maximise involvement across the sector, and the three-year timescale, meant that identification, evaluation and promotion activities were undertaken simultaneously, although for the purposes of this paper they have been treated sequentially.

A firm basis for identifying good practices was a project consortium with different backgrounds and expertise. On average, each project involved five consortium partners. Individual partners often took responsibility for different domains or sub-projects. Singly or jointly, many projects started in 1997/98 with a national survey, typically to gather data on numbers (official statistics from the Higher Education Statistics Agency (HESA) or the Universities and Colleges Admission Service (UCAS) are incomplete), on current practice and on perceived needs. Surveys were undertaken of residence abroad, of independent learning, of Internet use, of non-specialist provision, of staff training, of peer observation and of languages in art and design courses; many were repeated at a later stage in the project to evaluate change.

A further source of initial information was the published reports of the HEFCE QA process, which were analysed with respect to independent learning, assessment and residence abroad; for the latter, on-line summaries and a searchable database were made available. Dialogue with staff, whether academic, administrative or managerial, has been a feature of all projects and, although the FDTL projects are discipline-based, projects have also reached out to non-language staff, for example in staff development, student counselling, disability or careers. In addition to survey responses, projects have called upon feedback on websites, on-line discussion groups, use of existing mailbase lists, regional workshops, institutional visits and papers or workshop sessions at professional and research conferences. As an example, CIEL conducted 21 visits to individual universities, TransLang 19, RAPPORT 31 and ALLADIN 38.

Though not undertaken by all projects, dialogue with students has also been a major source of data, for example on experiences of residence abroad. The assessment project involved 176 students, Interculture more than 500, SMILE more than 500 and RAPPORT over 3000. Published reports have also contributed, including in some cases substantial research literature: it is worth noting that certain FDTL Languages project teams were already widely published and recognised for research expertise in areas including learner autonomy, residence abroad and intercultural communication. The research expertise has ensured that recommendations coming from the projects have a solid theoretical grounding as well as demonstrated practical effectiveness.

Workshops have nearly always led to written feedback and published reports, which are themselves key documents in establishing current practice and attitudes. Dialogue with staff and students has also accompanied the piloting of materials and methodologies to evaluate alternative approaches. Some projects have systematically used questionnaires, interviews and focus groups in their interactions with the sector, while synchronous (audio, video and computer conferencing) and asynchronous on-line discussion has been widespread. Examples of piloting include LARA's ethnographic training module for residence abroad, language learning strategy pack, academic cultural briefings, learning agreements and learner diaries; SMILE's computer conferencing in Italian, German and Dutch or the materials trialled by DEVELOP, DOPLA, ALLADIN or the assessment project.

A common approach to dissemination began even before funding was secured in 1997. Uniquely among FDTL projects, those in modern languages agreed in advance of the second round of bidding that they would co-operate in order to enhance dissemination. Impact would be maximised and nuisance to the sector minimised by the establishment of the Co-ordinating Group for Languages (FDTL-CGL). At its nine plenary meetings over three years, individual plans were discussed and joint activities scheduled – starting with a sharing of national surveys which reduced to five the number of questionnaires circulated to institutions at the launch of FDTL Languages. FDTL-CGL met at CILT, founded in 1966 to support language teachers at all levels, and the projects contracted CILT to provide a joint dissemination service. This comprised, as well as support for the CGL meetings:

- a single FDTL Languages information point;
- telephone enquiry service;
- shared visual identity;
- six newsletters between 1997 and 2000, totalling 22,000 copies;
- successive leaflets;
- conference folders;
- a booklet describing projects' research outcomes;
- a common FDTL Languages website which recorded in all, over two years, 25,000 hits, peaking appropriately in May 2000 at 800 hits a week, and recording interest from over 50 countries;
- an annual conference whose function and profile evolved as the projects progressed, and concluded with the international conference *The New Communicators: Graduates with Languages* in July 2000, attended by over 250 people.

As well as the common identity, projects developed their own visual identities, acronyms and logos and some issued their own regular newsletters and updates. Dissemination activities may be categorised on a four-point continuum from 'passive', via 'reactive' and 'semi-active' to 'active'. In the first 'passive' category are offerings which are simply made available, which inform those who make the effort to find them, and primary amongst these are project websites. Although they featured in many original bids, the importance they have attained testifies to the way FDTL Languages have responded to the evolution of ICT in educational contexts. While all provide project information, for WELL, DOPLA and RAPPORT the website has become a principal project output, providing thousands of files and links and attracting over 100 hits each week. It is my personal view that in education, change happens so fast these days that a dynamic means of dissemination is essential: printed outputs become out of date too quickly.

'Passive' dissemination must also include other outputs which potential end-users are under no pressure to engage with, such as newsletters, reports, leaflets and posters distributed via mailing lists, and assorted packs, booklets, videos and CD-ROMs. At the margins of this category in which dissemination depends on the user's volition are the scarlet sweatshirts with the RESIDENCE ABROAD MATTERS logo which many FDTL Languages participants will be unable to forget.

By 'reactive' dissemination I understand complementarity, arousing users' interest by offering something more than a leaflet or website or drawing them to the website by a related offer. LARA was the first project to run a competition (for student essays); like the later RAPPORT electronic postcard competition, the dissemination objective was achieved although the numbers of staff and student browsers whom the competition attracted outweighed the actual student entries. Interculture's comic postcards invited student responses but likewise lured all categories of users to the project website, as did everyone's conference and workshop presentations and the announcement of RAPPORT's accredited distance learning MA unit offering staff development in regard to supporting residence abroad. Also under the 'reactive' heading come telephone and Internet helplines and a range of on-line activities, from the WELL treasure hunt and on-line interactive workshops to the various searchable bibliographies and databases, including the extensive Interculture database of first-person student experiences while abroad.

'Semi-active' dissemination involves projects' going to the territory of end-users, whether by delivering conference papers, publishing in research journals, using existing e-mail networks, feeding articles to the press (local, national and professional), or exploiting horizontal links with subject associations, Computers in Teaching Initiative (CTI) centres or – occasionally – linking with FDTL projects in other disciplines. By mid-2000 Interculture, for instance, had given eleven conference papers and seen two articles published.

'Active' dissemination can be the most effective form, since target users participate actively in projects. The category includes FDTL Languages conferences and the very many themed workshops: ALLADIN ran 4, TransLang 5, DEVELOP 13 and the Residence Abroad Matters group 8, including a separate one for decision makers and quality assurance heads, with a different agenda from the practitioners' workshop. At the latter, active involvement was assured by the Residence Abroad Matters Game, an engaging simulation devised by LARA's Linda Parker involving real-life scenarios and resource-based decision making.

Site visits also proved effective for identification, evaluation, dissemination and training, providing a forum for staff from across an institution to focus on a single issue: more than once, they acted as a catalyst for changes in practice. Providing some funding for sub-projects, sometimes on a basis of competitive bids, helped DOPLA, LARA, WELL and Interculture to involve directly staff from other institutions. Accredited staff development has helped individual colleagues make a difference in their own department: examples include RAPPORT's on-line Supporting Residence Abroad unit, SMILE's training for language advisers, use of DOPLA materials in accredited teaching certificates and the citation of DEVELOP and other materials in successful applications for membership of the Institute for

Learning and Teaching in Higher Education (ILT), the new professional body whose mission is to raise the profile and prestige of effective university teaching.

Special mention should be made of accessibility. Additional funding was made available against successful bids to extend the outcomes of FDTL projects to those with a range of disabilities. Examples of successful applications include websites adapted for visual impairment or the work of SMILE, CIEL and ALLADIN to extend to dyslexic students the benefits of independent learning.

Such an enumeration of dissemination strategies invites a direct question: what works?

Despite the received wisdom that nobody reads newsletters, the contrary was demonstrated when a mention in a NCT newsletter for FDTL projects of a free meeting room in central London brought so many inquiries that the facility had to be withdrawn. However, the general conclusion among the projects is that newsletters and similar paper-based awareness raising are necessary but not sufficient. Paper-based questionnaires or websites which invited respondents to alert projects to examples of good practice proved much less effective than personal contacts, especially site visits. And as the earlier TLTP programme showed, the 'not invented here' syndrome embodies resistance to any materials or methods in whose development the sector as a whole has not participated.

Mailbase or Internet-based discussions proved excessively hard to prime and to maintain, even if carefully structured: WELL was the honourable exception. Even when subsidies were offered to departments to try new approaches, take-up and actual reports were sometimes thin on the ground, although DEVELOP, TransLang, LARA and WELL all supported informative case studies. Staff development carrying accreditation, however, by appealing to the individual's long-term career interests rather than to the department's short-term finances, was one strategy which demonstrably changed institutional practices.

Regrettably, since its existence was unique, no formal evaluation was carried out of the FDTL-CGL, but impartial observers were impressed by its openness and collaboration. It provides a possible model for the future and is indeed continuing in existence under the Learning and Teaching Support Network (LTSN) Subject Centre for Languages, Linguistics and Area Studies, whose co-operative network approach it may in part have inspired. Nonetheless, it has to be recognised that the FDTL-CGL did not succeed in eliminating overlap and duplication, that it could have done more to ensure experiences and dissemination techniques were shared and that it failed to persuade HEFCE that the LTSN Subject Centres – the third stage of active discipline-based quality enhancement following QA and FDTL – should adopt a distributed rather than an institution-based strategy.

And what are the actual outcomes or, in FDTL jargon, 'deliverables' of FDTL Languages? Some are finite – the innovative and effective paper-based, audio, video and CD-ROM materials of which every university languages department in the country has received a copy. Authoritative guides to language advising or managing the many facets of independent language learning or residence abroad now exist. There are evaluation reports in the public domain and the list of research publications will lengthen as project teams find proper time for analysis and writing up. As well as individual publications and the present volume born of the final FDTL Languages conference and co-sponsored by three other organisations, at least two edited book-length collections will draw heavily on FDTL Languages experience: *Training to teach languages in higher education* (ed. Klapper for CILT) and *Effective learning and teaching in modern languages* (ed. Coleman for ILT/Kogan Page).

Then there are the several comprehensive, interactive, dynamic websites, many of which will continue in existence thanks to continuation funding or, more properly, 'transferability' funding, since the money seeks to ensure the FDTL outcomes are taken on by the Subject Centre. Language advisers, now more numerous than in 1997, remain in post. New syllabuses and materials have been adopted. Site visits and regional workshops are continuing. Staff development using FDTL Languages materials continues on a national scale and websites are set to be exploited more fully, not least the DOPLA site at Birmingham University since project co-ordinator John Klapper has been named as one of the first twenty National Teaching Fellows. The combined potential of the FDTL Languages websites as a national resource will, it is hoped, be fully realised as they are brought still closer together under the umbrella of the Subject Centre. The latter's existence constitutes an acceptance that continuity is preferable to short-term projects and that quality is often best enhanced, and professional staff development managed, through discipline-based initiatives rather than the traditional generic approach. Too many staff developers in the past have derided subject-specific approaches – 'every subject thinks it's different' – before implementing, at institutional and national level, generic programmes which individual university staff, with their discipline-based identity and loyalty, have consistently ignored. Additionally, since the subject community will now define needs and priorities, the quality agenda should be more inclusive than was the case for FDTL Languages.

There has also been an international impact beyond the hits recorded on the FDTL Languages website: we can point for example to the conferences and publications of the European Language Council; to SMILE workshops in Germany, Finland, Italy and Greece; to CIEL in Ireland and Germany; to interest in DOPLA from Ireland, France and South Africa and in DEVELOP not just in Europe but from Japan and Indonesia; to RAPPORT links in the USA. Bids are already in to extend positive

FDTL outcomes across Europe and there is clear scope for British higher education to build on such initiatives and contribute its expertise to worldwide discussion of enhancing quality in university learning.

So, have FDTL Languages really brought about changes? Where is the hard evidence of two million pounds' worth of impact? Under the influence of SMILE, the number of language adviser posts has increased from 7 to 35. There now exist accredited undergraduate modules on independent language learning, study skills, presentation skills and ICT and tandem learning. Changes have been made to art and design courses, to residence abroad assessment, to the training of foreign language assistants and postgraduates, to staff tandem observation. We can show conclusively that every higher education institution in the country offering language courses has participated in FDTL Languages activities and that few if any modern languages staff are unaware of the projects and their outcomes – but individuals remain entitled to ignore all the FDTL work, as long as they remain persuaded that the return on their effort is many times higher for research than it is for learning and teaching activities.

It will always be hard to demonstrate a single cause for change, especially until all the project evaluations and comparative surveys are complete. The real proof will be long term and first measured in the Quality Assurance Agency reviews of languages to take place in 2003–6. The new methods adopted to review academic quality and standards refer explicitly to 'external reference points', to 'sharing best practice', and to 'previous subject reviews'; and whatever individual academics choose to prioritise, UK institutions cannot ignore either the good practices and problem issues raised in the 1995/96 QA process, or the FDTL Languages' efforts to promote the former and address the latter.

Through their intensive programme of surveys, workshops, websites, newsletters, conferences and institutional visits, the FDTL Languages projects have been seeking to identify, describe, disseminate and promote best practice in their respective domains. All the stake-holders – government, parents, students, employers and institutions themselves – now have benchmarks against which the procedures and performance of any individual institution can be measured.

References

Bradbeer, J. (2000) *The experience of staff and educational development*, University of Portsmouth (Occasional Paper No. 2 of FDTL Project Integrating People and Technology).

Coleman, J. A. and Parker, G. (1992) *French and the enterprise path: developing transferable and professional skills.* London: AFLS/Centre for Information on Language Teaching and Research.

Coleman, J. A. (1996) *Studying languages: a survey of British and European students. The proficiency, background, attitudes and motivations of students of foreign languages in the United Kingdom and Europe.* London: Centre for Information on Language Teaching and Research.

Evans, C. (1988) *Language people.* Open University Press.

HEFCE (1996) *Overview reports for French* (QO 2/96), *German and related languages* (QO 3/96), *Iberian languages and studies* (QO 4/96), *Italian* (QO 5/96), *Russian* (QO7/96). Available at www.qaa.ac.uk/revreps/subjrev/bysubname.htm

McKeachie, W. J. (1997) Critical elements in training university teachers, *International Journal for Academic Development,* 2 (1): 67–74.

The Nuffield Languages Inquiry (2000) *Languages: the next generation.* London: Nuffield Foundation.

Towell, R. J. (1998) Higher Education, in Moys A., (ed) *Where are we going with languages?* London: Nuffield Foundation: 46–54.

Residence abroad and the learning process: redefining the objectives

Mark Bannister ◉ *Oxford Brookes University*

In terms of learning and teaching, the period of residence abroad, which forms an essential part of the great majority of first degrees in modern languages, is uniquely anomalous. Students are enrolled in a department in the UK but are not present in it. They are required to carry out certain academic tasks or to follow certain courses abroad which have been neither designed nor validated by the department and which it does not deliver or control. Alternatively, they may be required to take up work in an office or school which may well have little to do with what they are studying in the department.

The difficulties of ensuring that the learning process while abroad is integrated with the curricular progression on which the rest of the course is based are considerable and most departments have had little success in that area, as the overview reports produced at the end of the Teaching Quality Assessment round in 1995–96 made clear. Nearly 70% of German departments had not integrated the period abroad well into the rest of the curriculum or established clear objectives for it. Again, in French, about 70% of providers had not successfully integrated the period abroad into the curriculum. In Iberian languages, 'many institutions were criticised for their lack of design, planning, operation and evaluation of the period abroad and its place within the curriculum as a whole', with 'the aims and objectives of the period abroad not fully identified and explained to the students' and 'a virtual absence of significant curricular integration and accreditation links with foreign institutions'. In Italian, less successful practice (indicated as being usually found among the larger providers) was characterised by 'lack of clear objectives [...] and a lack of awareness of how the experience [of residence abroad] could be used to enhance the students' performance in other parts of the programme'.

Despite all the effort and goodwill put in by departments, there is clearly a problem area here, the solution to which arguably involves rethinking the academic and educational objectives of the period abroad and identifying the elements that would, ideally, permit a seamless progression throughout the four years of the degree-course. That in its turn requires a consideration of the methods of learning adopted by students, the ways in which they set goals for themselves and the structure of the learning process itself.

In the 1970s, there was much discussion amongst educational psychologists of a classification of students' approaches to learning into 'deep' and 'surface', the 'deep' approach being concerned to extract the underlying meaning from a text or similar piece of work and the structures built into it, the 'surface' approach being content to remain at the level of memorising or reproducing (Säljö, 1975, Svensson, 1976, Marton, 1979). Subsequent research by Ramsden, Biggs and others offered modifications of this classification (division of both 'deep' and 'surface' approaches into 'active' and 'passive'; addition of a third 'strategic' approach), but one of the key conclusions to emerge was a strong correlation between the students' approach to learning and their conception of learning: two thirds of those who used a 'deep' approach saw learning as the abstraction of meaning or as an interpretative process aimed at understanding reality (Ramsden, 1988, Biggs, 1993). The inference is that students in higher education, who are expected to be able to interact actively and critically with the ideas they meet, should be encouraged to adopt a 'deep' approach. There is no agreement as to whether all students are capable of adopting a 'deep' approach, but Graham Gibbs has shown that a 'surface' approach is more common in departments where the class-contact hours are high, where there is an excessive amount of course material and where the students do not have the opportunity to pursue subjects in depth, which suggests that changes to learning and teaching strategies can produce significant improvements in terms of learning outcomes (Gibbs, 1992).

In 1988, Ames and Archer identified two different goal orientations in learners: 'mastery' and 'performance'. Those who adopted 'mastery' goals were more likely to be intrinsically motivated, choose more challenging tasks and persist for longer, link their own academic success and failure to the amount of effort they expended and the strategies they used and value learning for its own sake. In contrast, those with a 'performance' goal orientation were more likely to be extrinsically motivated, choose tasks which they knew they could achieve easily and link academic success and failure to ability, and be less concerned with learning *per se* than with preserving their self-image as competent individuals (Ames and Archer, 1988). A good deal of effort has gone into investigating whether it is possible to promote the adoption of 'mastery' goals and one important area that is held to be crucial is the link between perceived learning autonomy and intrinsic motivation. If students feel that they are responsible for the outcomes of their own learning, they are more likely to adopt 'mastery' goals, putting in more effort, choosing more challenging tasks, developing strategies appropriate to the task and the context. Learning autonomy does not, of course, mean being left entirely to one's own devices. There has to be a framework within which self-determination can be exercised and, in an educational context, that framework is set by the curriculum and the requirements of the particular course.

In the 1990s, the schema-theory of learning aroused much interest (see Desforges, 1998). A schema is defined as a person's organised experience in reference to a specific context or setting. The schema is constantly being modified by a process of accretion, tuning, restructuring. Accretion is the acquisition of new items of knowledge or new associations. Tuning, which is often subconscious, involves the cutting out of redundant stages in the comprehension process. Restructuring, as the word implies, is the re-ordering of the schema to embody the new insights. The schema-theory has the great advantage of looking at the learning process from the internal point of view (inside the student's mind), regardless of how the knowledge is acquired or has been presented from outside. It is therefore arguably of particular relevance to learning during a period abroad, in which the student is in a permanent learning situation as regards the language and culture.

A number of caveats need to be formulated at this point. Much of the work outlined above was carried out largely in the context of classroom-based or book-based learning, which is less immediately relevant to the experience of the period abroad. Some of it concerns secondary rather than higher education, which again may make it less relevant. None the less, it is legitimate to look for ways of designing a period abroad experience which encourages 'deep' rather than 'surface' learning, puts a premium on 'mastery' goal orientation and ensures that the process of 'tuning' and 'restructuring' the schema takes place as efficiently as possible.

As was suggested above, the period abroad is anomalous in terms of the learning and teaching process as it is normally carried out in British higher education, viz a process prescribed and controlled by the staff in the home department, designed on a sequential and progressive basis, involving a mixture of classroom and self-directed learning, with assessment and accreditation carried out by the home department. It is certainly possible to approximate to that pattern during the period abroad by finding a university where the students can follow courses that are passably similar to those at home and by agreeing with the staff there how the students will be taught and assessed. To a certain extent, it is possible to cater for the self-directed learning aspect by requiring the students to carry out a project or write a dissertation based on material drawn from the context in which they are living, which can then be assessed and accredited by the home department. However, as language staff are well aware, the reality is never more than an approximation to the desired curriculum, which is why there is almost universal reluctance to treat the period abroad (almost always an academic year) as a fully recognised part of the learning process and to give it the full academic credit it deserves.

In any rethinking of the objectives of the period abroad, the starting-point ought to be the one factor that differentiates it from the rest of the course, the fact that the students are immersed for a substantial period in the language and culture they are studying. That great resource is, of course, recognised by most departments, at least in theory. Over 90% of them say the primary objectives of the period abroad are that the students should improve their linguistic competence and their intercultural understanding.[1] But it is generally assumed that it will happen by osmosis, just by hearing the language and experiencing the culture.

Schema-theory might seem at first sight to give some support to the osmotic approach. As regards accretion, the students are constantly acquiring new items of knowledge. There ought, too, to be a speeding up of the understanding process, i.e. 'tuning'. When it comes to restructuring and the creation of new insights, however, there is a strong likelihood that, rather than gaining new insights, they would simply be confirming the stereotypes with which they arrived. And the osmotic approach will certainly not facilitate 'deep' learning or 'mastery' goal orientation.

In the light of what language departments are trying or hoping to achieve, what they actually require of students during the period abroad and what they perceive to be the problematic aspects of the residence-abroad experience, we can conclude:

a. that the process of autonomous learning, which many departments would acknowledge as desirable throughout the degree course, must be absolutely central to the period abroad;

b. that that process must be principally applied to the primary objectives of the period abroad, i.e. improvement in linguistic competence and intercultural understanding.

Autonomous learning, where the students are ultimately in charge of the process that leads to their achieving specified objectives, is more likely to encourage deep learning, more conducive to the adoption of 'mastery' goals, more appropriate for bringing about the restructuring of schemas to embody valid new insights.

However, there are a number of important corollaries. First, the students cannot simply be told to go away and learn autonomously, although that is basically what the osmotic approach assumes: autonomy is not the same as total independence. They have to be trained in the methods they will need to apply while they are abroad, so that they know how to exercise genuine control over their own learning. Secondly, it is essential that the students have specific goals so that they know what exactly their learning skills are going to be used for and what they will be expected to have achieved. Thirdly, the students' motivation has to be maintained by ensuring that the achievement of the outcomes of the period abroad is assessed on more than a pass/fail basis and that the marks they receive are properly accredited within the degree programme as a whole.

The conversion of these principles into practical experience depends on the development of new attitudes which will have an impact on the assumptions made about the activities undertaken by the students. Both students and staff will come to appreciate that the learning that counts while the students are abroad goes on all the time and is not necessarily dependent on the 'day-job', which usually involves following courses or working in an office or school. It will certainly be taking place during those activities, but it will equally be going on in all sorts of unofficial and social situations, at weekends, in families, in cafés and clubs, and so on. Such situations are the raw material on which the students exercise the observational, analytical and deductive skills in which they have been trained. For that reason, the training in autonomous learning methods has to be treated seriously. It cannot be imparted simply in an hour or two of a preparatory session at the end of the year before the period abroad. It needs to be integrated into the teaching programme for at least a semester before the students go abroad and, again, integrated with the work they do after their return. After all, degree courses are designed on the assumption that the acquisition and exercise of intellectual skills, the effectiveness of which is measured at the end of the course in a number of outcomes, go on for three years and are assumed to be embedded in all the academic activities undertaken by the students.

What, then, does the training need to consist of? The language course that students follow in the year before they go abroad should contain a significant element showing the students how to develop their own learning strategies for exploiting the whole range of language-learning opportunities with which their new environment will provide them. They will find themselves in a vast 'resource centre' and they will need to know, for example, how to be proactive in building up their lexical base, how to distinguish a range of registers and levels and apply them appropriately, how to apply the knowledge that written language is not just spoken language written down. These skills are best taught, not in the abstract and in isolation, but through the carrying out of tasks, learning from practical situations, embedded into the language course that every degree programme includes in each year.

On the intercultural side, it is particularly difficult for the students to make sense of the 'resource centre' represented by the foreign culture if they have not been trained in how to exploit it. The exhortations commonly given to students to 'develop an intelligent approach to what is going on around you at all levels of your daily life' or to be 'open-minded and receptive' will not help beyond the observational level. Any real understanding has to start from a solid basis of awareness that 'culture' is not a monolithic set of practices or attitudes common to a nation, but a constantly changing set of patterns of interaction arising out of ideological and axiological assumptions, very often unconscious; that language and culture are inextricably linked; that there is no justification for thinking that any one type of behaviour is 'normal' or 'natural'; and that intercultural learning is ultimately about investigating, in an intellectual and rigorous way, the phenomenon of 'otherness'. If intellectual rigour is to be maintained and the learning process during the period abroad is to be the equal of that expected in the rest of the course, the students need to be able to investigate in detail an aspect of the society in which they find themselves, having learned how to observe and assemble evidence, how to interpret, how to draw valid conclusions. They need, in short, to be taught the essentials of ethnography and shown how to practise their skills in real situations.

A good deal of innovative work has been going on across the sector in terms of improving the effectiveness of language training for the period abroad. Ethnography, on the other hand, is not a discipline in which most staff in language departments have any expertise. However, those interested in pursuing the approach proposed in this article can avail themselves of the materials published by the Learning and Residence Abroad (LARA) project during the summer of 2000.[2] They include a pack containing a series of Language Tasks and Strategies for Students Abroad which encourage the students to focus on their own language progress by undertaking guided tasks relating to their everyday experiences, and an ethnography programme, including a module 'Introduction to Ethnography' based on anthropological concepts and fieldwork, which provides intellectual and practical experience in cultural and intercultural learning.

If the objectives of the period abroad are redefined in the way proposed, with the emphasis shifted from the primary activity to the learning process, a number of benefits should ensue. The students are less likely to retreat into 'ex-pat' or 'tourist' mode, because the onus is on them to go out and communicate with the locals. It should be easier to find a standard form of assessment for all students, whether they are on a study placement or a work placement, because the expected outcomes are the same for all of them. The students will be engaged in an intellectually and academically demanding programme validated by the home department, even though they may be spending the day carrying out mindless tasks in an office. They will come to appreciate, from first-hand experience, how language and culture are interlocked, which has implications for most other aspects of their degree course. And being responsible for their own learning is likely to have a psychological spin-off in terms of improving their self-confidence, sense of initiative and interpersonal skills, which is seen by most departments as an important secondary outcome of residence abroad.

Changes to the way in which the learning process is approached assume a corresponding change in the method of assessment and accreditation applied to the period abroad. If the students are, to a large extent, taking responsibility for their own learning, the process can be taken into account as well as the outcomes. An individual learning agreement, in which a set of personal objectives for the student is laid out, can not only indicate the formal requirements, e.g. completion of an ethnographic project, but can also help to track the less tangible benefits, such as the development of personal skills and qualities. If such things are included in the learning agreement and the student is monitoring their development, they will be taken more seriously than is usually the case. The ultimate goal might well be to have such a complete appraisal of the outcomes of the period abroad – linguistic, intercultural and personal – that it attracts the same amount of credit in the final degree assessment as any of the other years or corresponding periods.

A common response from hard-pressed staff concerned with residence abroad is to protest that such changes would represent an extra layer of work for both students and staff, not only during the period abroad but throughout the rest of the course as well, for which resources are not available. It is true that making the transition itself would require some extra work but, in the longer term, what is involved is not the input of extra resources so much as the redeployment of existing teaching resources. For instance, the year or semester before the students go abroad invariably includes a compulsory language module or course unit. That module needs to be **redrafted** to teach the students how to take charge of their own learning, but no extra resources would be needed. Similarly, there is likely to be another module or course-unit dealing with the contemporary state of the country in question, covering aspects of the national culture or mentality, and that module could be **replaced** by an introduction to ethnography or, at the least, **modified** to include training in intercultural awareness. Training in ethnographical methodology is not an alien intrusion into a language degree but supports every other academic aspect of the course and should be very much in line with its intellectual aims. Again, while the students are actually abroad, the assessed work required of them, and certainly that which is accredited, is, in a large number of cases, set and marked by the staff in the home department. It often takes the form of a dissertation or project which the staff have to mark. Marking an ethnographical or intercultural project instead is not going to produce extra work. In those cases where the students are on a SOCRATES exchange and are required to pass every element in a set programme in order to achieve full credit at the home institution, there may be a problem in requiring further work from them, but such cases seem to be a minority.

The period of residence abroad is an essential part of any degree course that includes the acquisition of a detailed knowledge of a foreign language and culture: its worth has been proved over several decades. However, in the present climate, when value for money quite rightly has to be demonstrated and the time spent on various activities justified, it must be shown to provide academic and educational outcomes of at least equal value to those of the rest of the course. As has been argued here, that means shifting the emphasis from the formal activities required of the students to the process of learning, taking full advantage of the linguistic and cultural environment in which they find themselves. Different departments operate in different ways with different aims, different structures and different traditions, and there will therefore be different solutions. The important thing is to rethink and re-establish the objectives and find the best ways of fulfilling them.

Notes

1 As shown in the questionnaire survey carried out in 1997/98 for the National Residence Abroad Database.
2 See http://lara.fdtl.ac.uk/lara/index.htm for an outline of the materials and contact details.

References

Ames, C. and Archer, J. (1988) 'Achievement goals in the classroom: students' learning strategies and motivation processes' in *Journal of Educational Psychology* 80 (3): 260–67.

Biggs, J. B. and Moore, P. J. (1993) *The process of learning*. Prentice Hall.

Deci, E. R. and Ryan, R. M. (1985) *Intrinsic motivation and self-determination in human behaviour*. Plenum Press.

Desforges, C. (1998) 'Learning and teaching: current views and perspectives' in Shorrocks-Taylor, D. (ed) *Directions in educational psychology*. Whurr.

Gibbs, G. (1992) *Improving the quality of student learning*. Technical and Educational Services.

Marton, F. (1979) *Learning as seen from the learner's point of view*. ERIC.

Ramsden, P. (ed) (1988) *Improving learning: new perspectives*. Kogan Page.

Säljö, R. (1975) *Qualitative differences in learning as a function of the learner's conception of the task*. Abacus.

Svensson, L. (1976) *Study skill and learning*. Acta Universitatis Gothenburgensis.

How independent can independent language learning really be?

David Little • Trinity College, Dublin

1 Introduction

For the purposes of this paper I shall use the term *independent language learning* to refer to learning that is undertaken independently of the direct control of a teacher. Sometimes it supplements classroom learning; sometimes it constitutes a total approach; in universities it is usually supported by the kind of technical installations one associates with language centres – language laboratories, video playback, satellite television and multimedia computers with Internet access.

The concept of independent language learning in this sense arose several decades ago from the realization that language laboratories could be used not only for class teaching but by students working on their own. Used in this way, the language laboratory offered to fulfil much the same function for language learning as the library had long fulfilled for other forms of learning. It was thus not surprising that when universities began to set up language centres the language laboratory generally served as the foundation stone. Inevitably, some language centres were viewed with suspicion by the foreign language departments they were supposed to serve. In the case of my own centre, the suspicion was strong enough to ban us from language teaching for many years, and this left us with no alternative but to promote the idea of independent learning and develop various self-access programmes. Even without this kind of political pressure, language centres have been attracted to independent learning as something that offers to give them a distinctive character, in principle complementary to, but undeniably different from, the language-teaching activity of the traditional foreign language department.

From the beginning proponents of independent language learning have been concerned to identify the skills that students need in order to achieve independent learning success. Typically these skills have been described in relation to the concept of learner autonomy, which has often been understood as another term for learner independence. The obvious fact that large numbers of students do not possess independent learning skills has made it necessary to devise means of stimulating their growth. In particular, learner counselling has emerged as a distinctive form of pedagogical intervention. Nevertheless, schemes of independent learning all too often remain worryingly recalcitrant; too often there seems to be something fundamentally wrong or lacking. Increasingly my own efforts to theorize the concept of learner autonomy have prompted me to ask the question that provides the title for this paper. I shall answer it first by offering some reflections on the nature of human learning and the concept of learner autonomy and then by considering various modes of independent language learning from the perspective thus established.

2 Human learning and the concept of learner autonomy

2.1 A *social-interactive view of learning*

Social interaction plays an indispensable role in human learning. At first sight this statement may seem to be no more than a truism. Learning is, after all, a matter of acquiring knowledge and/or skills that we do not already possess and the most obvious means of acquisition is via socially mediated processes of communication. In Western societies children typically grow up in nuclear families that belong to extended families and are connected to larger communities in many different ways; and schools, colleges and universities are social organizations in their own right.

But a social-interactive view of learning does not simply propose that learning is socially mediated: it claims that learning arises from a complex interplay between individual-cognitive and social-interactive processes. In doing so it gives equal importance to two basic facts about the human organism. On the one hand each of us is a self-contained, *autopoietic* being (Maturana and Varela, 1987). We develop, cognitively as well as physically, according to laws that are written in our genes, and our consciousness in all its complexity is entirely private to ourselves. Outside agencies cannot determine the course or speed of our biological development and they cannot gain direct access to our thoughts. In that sense we cannot help but be autonomous. On the other hand, we are social creatures who depend on one another in a multitude of ways and our development proceeds in complex interaction with a multitude of environmental factors and constraints. Without socialization, for example, children cannot acquire a mother tongue and without socialization they cannot develop the 'theory of mind' (e.g. Astington, 1994) which enables them to grasp from a very early age that, like them, other people have thoughts and emotions, beliefs and desires.

A sense that it is ultimately impossible to separate these two dimensions of human nature underlies those theories of cognition and learning that emphasize the interdependence of the individual-cognitive and the social-interactive. Perhaps the most influential of these theories for work on child development, but also for the psychology of education, has been that of Lev Vygotsky (1978, 1986), for whom the higher cognitive functions were the product of social interaction. Vygotsky saw this as 'the distinguishing feature of human psychology, the basis of the qualitative leap from animal to human psychology' (Vygotsky, 1978: 57). According to this view, learning is the product of supported performance – the 'zone of proximal development', for which Vygotsky is perhaps best known in educational circles, is

> the distance between the actual developmental level as determined by independent problem solving and the level of potential development as determined through problem solving under adult guidance or in collaboration with more capable peers. (1978: 86)

Other theories of cognition similarly emphasize the inescapable dependence of the individual-cognitive on the social-interactive. One thinks, for example, of such notions as 'distributed cognition', which seeks to account for the fact that we 'appear to think in conjunction or partnership with others and with the help of culturally provided tools and implements' (Salomon, 1993: xiii); 'situated learning' (Lave and Wenger, 1991, Wenger, 1998), which is concerned with the fact that we learn by constructing meanings and identities as members of 'communities of practice'; and 'interactive minds', which 'implies that the acquisition and manifestation of individual cognitions influence and are influenced by cognitions of others' (Baltes and Staudinger, 1996: 6).

In stressing the importance of the social-interactive dimension of cognition and learning, it is important not to underplay the importance of the individual-cognitive dimension. As Ackermann (1996: 32) puts it:

> Without connection people cannot grow, yet without separation they cannot relate.
>
> People cannot learn from their experience as long as they are entirely immersed in it. There comes a time when they need to step back, and from a distance reconsider what has happened to them. They must take on the role of an external observer, or critic, and they must revisit their experience 'as if' it were not theirs. They need to describe it to themselves and others, and in doing so, they will make it tangible. (ibid: 28)

This thought leads Ackermann to represent cognitive growth, but also learning, as 'a dance between diving in and stepping out' (ibid). The truth of this metaphor is confirmed by early child development. Social interaction is essential to first language acquisition – without socially framed talk, linguistic development is impossible; but no less essential is the time that the child spends alone, talking to herself, playing with words, assisting the internalization process by rehearsal and language games (Crystal, 1999: 166). The second of these dimensions of child development apparently depends on the first for its shape and content: the child's spoken thoughts seem to take their impetus from the experience of saying and doing in interaction with others (for a sustained case study with far-reaching implications, see Nelson, 1989). In other words, patterns of verbal thinking are determined by the structures of interactive discourse. Much the same insight underpins studies of the language of early schooling that emphasize the importance of establishing links between classroom discourse and the discourse of the home (see, e.g., Tizard and Hughes, 1984, Wells, 1987).

The argument so far carries two important implications, one for independent learning in general and one for independent language learning in particular. If social interaction is essential to child development as the paradigm case of human learning, it follows that independent learning in the sense of self-instruction will succeed to the extent that the learner has a developed capacity to internalize social interaction as psychological process. And if the acquisition of a mother tongue arises in part from the fact that language is the tool by which we shape and control social interaction, we must ask how far independent language learning will be able to go when learners are deprived of the necessity to interact in the target language even as they attempt to learn it. The practical examples I shall present and discuss later in my paper will bring us back to these considerations, but first it is necessary to ask ourselves how learner autonomy fits into the picture.

2.2   *Learner autonomy and independent learning*

By *autonomy* I mean a capacity for self-motivated and self-regulated behaviour. In this sense, autonomy is the biological goal of child development and the social goal of most parenting: children count as mature when they are able to make their own decisions and accept responsibility for the outcomes of their own behaviour. As any parent knows, the extent to which children achieve this goal is infinitely variable, and it is clear that most of us retain some significant areas of helplessness throughout our lives.

Autonomy as a capacity for self-motivated and self-regulated behaviour is also the logical and often the declared goal of formal learning within educational systems. After all, long-term success in any school or university subject is a function of the extent to which the individual learner can apply the knowledge and skills he or she has learnt in the classroom to situations in the world outside the classroom and that can happen only on the basis of self-motivation and self-regulation. Some learners will always find their own way to autonomy, whatever pedagogical approach they are exposed to. But because formal learning is shaped by conscious intentions and explicit plans, the pursuit of autonomy in formal learning environments must entail explicit, conscious processes; otherwise we leave its development to chance.

Writing from the perspective of social-psychological research into human motivation, Deci (1996: 2) defines autonomy as follows:

> *To be autonomous means to act in accord with one's self – it means feeling free and volitional in one's actions. When autonomous, people are fully willing to do what they are doing, and they embrace the activity with a sense of interest and commitment. Their actions emanate from their true sense of self, so they are being authentic.*

According to Deci, autonomy is one of three innate psychological needs that all human beings experience, the others being competence and relatedness. We need to feel that we are behaving in the way we want to behave (autonomy) and that in doing so we are exploiting our developed proficiency (competence) and relating appropriately to the others with whom we are cast together (relatedness). The freedom that autonomy always entails is thus necessarily constrained by our social relationships and obligations. Clearly, this understanding of autonomy is a close relative of the social-interactive theories of cognition and learning that I have briefly reviewed.

In my introduction I noted that in discussion of independent language learning, autonomy is often assumed to be the same thing as independence. Deci, however, makes the following important distinction:

> *Independence means to do for yourself, to **not** rely on others for personal nourishment and emotional support. Autonomy, in contrast, means to act freely, with a sense of volition and choice. It is thus possible for a person to be independent and autonomous (i.e., to freely not rely on others), or to be independent and controlled (i.e., to feel forced not to rely on others).* (Deci, 1996: 89)

This distinction helps to explain why some of the most successful projects to develop learner autonomy have been conducted by teachers in classrooms, and on the other hand why many students enrolled in independent learning programmes fail to display truly autonomous behaviour.

In foreign language learning, autonomy has to do with learning but also with using the target language. I have argued elsewhere (Little, 1999) that its development depends on the operationalization of three principles. The first is the principle of **learner empowerment**: learners must be given responsibility for their own learning and its outcomes, which entails that they must be granted a share in the social control of the learning environment. The second is the principle of **target language use**: as far as possible the target language must be the medium as well as the goal of learning, for only thus can learners begin to develop spontaneous fluency and turn the target language into an instrument of thought. The third is the principle of **reflectivity**: learners must develop the capacity to engage in the reflective processes of planning, monitoring and evaluating their learning, for only thus can their learning be truly self-regulated.

Note that each of these principles requires the development of procedural skills. This fact has important implications for our understanding of how autonomy develops: essentially, the only way of becoming autonomous is to be autonomous. Note also that according to this view, the pursuit of autonomy engages the learner's intrinsic motivation and stimulates reflectivity. In other words, the development of learner autonomy brings the motivational and metacognitive dimensions of learning into interaction with each other. In all of this, of course, social interaction plays an indispensable role, so that when we turn our attention to the development of student autonomy in independent language-learning schemes, we are again confronted with the question: how do we provide for the social-interactive dimension of learning?

3 The practice of independent language learning

Having sketched a view of learning that emphasises the interdependence of social-interactive and individual-cognitive dimensions and defined learner autonomy as something different from learner independence, I shall now consider independent language learning in three different modes: first as a support for language classes, then as a total approach to language learning and finally in the form of tandem language learning via the Internet.

3.1 *Independent learning as a support for language classes*

Independent learning is central to our educational traditions: it has always been recognised that learners need to spend time on their own, consolidating and supplementing the learning that they do in classrooms. Yet homework is all too often discontinuous with what goes on in the classroom, so that learners are at a loss to know how to go about the task they have been given. Much the same can be said of the way in which students from the various language departments in Trinity College Dublin have tended to use the self-access facilities and resources in the Centre for Language and Communication Studies (CLCS). Several years ago my colleague Barbara Lazenby Simpson surveyed students' independent learning behaviour in our self-access centre (Lazenby Simpson, 1997). She confirmed what we already knew from informal observation: that our clients' favourite activity was watching pre-recorded videos or satellite television. She also confirmed what we suspected: that very few of them did so with any particular learning intention in mind. They mostly worked on the assumption that if they exposed themselves passively to their target language, some of it would somehow rub off on them. When asked what they thought they were likely to learn from watching videos or satellite television, they often gave implausible answers. Their passive and unfocused learning behaviour was no doubt connected with the fact that it was not continuous with what they did in their language classes, also with the fact that in their language classes they were not required to plan, monitor and evaluate their own learning. The lesson that Lazenby Simpson's study teaches is that if independent work is to support classroom learning, the two must be very thoroughly integrated. Learners cannot reasonably be expected to manage independent learning if they are not first involved in the management of classroom learning.

We were given an opportunity to attempt a thoroughgoing integration of independent with classroom learning some six years ago, when CLCS was made responsible for Trinity College's institution-wide language-learning programme (for a full account of the design and implementation of the programme, see Little and Ushioda, 1998). Essentially, we set out to devise a course structure that would impel students towards greater autonomy by operationalizing the three principles of learner empowerment, target language use and reflectivity. We built our courses on a series of four-week cycles in which students work in groups of four or five on projects of their own devising in their target language. At the end of each cycle projects are presented to the rest of the class. Within this programme students' use of our self-access facilities is very thoroughly determined by classroom work. In particular they use the Internet and various kinds of reference materials on CD-ROM to find information and textual examples relevant to the project under preparation. Nevertheless, given that these language courses are extra-curricular and our students have little time to devote to language learning, developing the kind of reflective approach to learning that is essential for the growth of learner autonomy has been an uphill struggle.

In the last two years, however, we have been able to apply our project-based approach to the design of two-year French and German modules that are an obligatory component of a new degree course in Information and Communications Technology. The fact that we have been piloting a version of the Council of Europe's European Language Portfolio (ELP) has added an extra dimension to this programme. The ELP comprises (i) a passport that summarizes the learner's linguistic identity, (ii) a language biography that records language-learning goals and significant learning and intercultural experiences and (iii) a dossier in which the learner keeps examples of his or her work. It is proving highly effective in helping students to develop a reflective and self-managing approach to their language learning. But again students' capacity to use the ELP as an individual tool for the management of language learning depends on the social-interactive mediation of appropriate techniques of planning, monitoring and evaluation. (CLCS's version of the ELP can be viewed at our website www.tcd.ie/CLCS/ and downloaded as a Word document file.)

3.2   *Independent language learning as a total approach*

Mention of the European Language Portfolio provides an appropriate transition to independent learning as a total approach. For success here depends on either recruiting learners who are already able to plan, monitor and evaluate their own learning or else helping learners who cannot yet do this to develop the necessary skills. That means engaging in exactly those reflective processes that the ELP is designed to promote.

The most interesting experiment I am aware of in this form of independent language learning is the Autonomous Learning Modules (ALMS) project of the Helsinki University Language Centre, reported on by Karlsson *et al* (1997). Interestingly, this project seems to have taken its first impetus from the need to save money, though that was essentially coincidental to the chief pedagogical focus of the project, which was on learning how to learn. The leaders of the project began by assuming that learner autonomy is a capacity that has to be consciously developed, which means that its pursuit entails a focus on process before product. They recognized that the development of learner autonomy has a social-interactive as well as an individual-cognitive dimension and that it calls for a change in the power structures of the learning environment as well as steady growth in learners' awareness of language-learning processes. They also recognised that the capacity for autonomous learning behaviour is unstable and vulnerable. Accordingly, it requires constant support and its implementation must take account of the particularities of socio-cultural context.

Let me briefly summarize how the ALMS project works in practice. At the beginning of each ALMS cycle (courses last one semester) there is a compulsory six-hour workshop designed to raise learners' awareness of language-learning processes and of themselves as language learners. This is followed by a compulsory three-hour workshop in which learners explore their needs and draw up learning contracts. These may focus on an individual programme of learning or a collaborative enterprise that involves one or more other learners. Undoubtedly the success of the project is due in no small measure to the amount of time that is spent at the beginning on interactive reflection, on using social interaction to stimulate appropriately focused individual cognition. According to Karlsson *et al* (1997), this is indispensable, for although Finnish students often come to university with a very good level of proficiency in foreign languages, their classroom experience has usually been of a traditional kind, which means that they have as much difficulty in coming to terms with the demands of independent learning as students in other countries. Once they embark on their programme of learning, they are supported by regular seminars in which they report on progress and explore problems. In the course of the term they are required to attend three 15-minute individual counselling sessions, which pick up on issues raised in the workshops at the beginning of term. In the ALMS project individual learning effort is always firmly embedded in social interaction.

3.3   Tandem language learning via e-mail and in the MOO

When applied to language learning, Ackermann's (1996: 28) 'dance between diving in and stepping out' implies an alternation between learning by doing and learning by analysis, between learning by performing communicative tasks and learning by reflecting on the target language and/or the language learning process. Now it has never been the case that independent learning activities can belong only to the 'stepping out' category. Reading, for example, is mostly a solitary activity and thus highly appropriate for independent learning, but it is an activity that requires us to **dive in** before we can **step out**. Nevertheless, it is probably true to say that historically most materials and activities designed for use in independent language learning have been detached from communicative interaction and thus biased towards 'stepping out'. In the last few years this situation has changed dramatically, thanks to the evolution of computer-mediated communication. In this section of my paper I shall focus on tandem language learning via e-mail and the MOO (Multiple-user domain, Object Oriented) because, despite sometimes formidable obstacles to implementation, these modes of learning combine communicative language use with an explicit and reflective concern with learning. In other words, they alternate between 'diving in' and 'stepping out' in a potentially very fruitful way.

Tandem language learning has been defined as a form of open learning in which two people with different native languages work together to learn one another's language, to learn more about one another's culture, and perhaps to exchange additional information (see Little and Brammerts, 1996: 10). It is constituted by the principles of reciprocity and autonomy. According to the principle of reciprocity, tandem learners must be equally committed to their own and their partner's language learning; this entails bilingual communication. According to the principle of autonomy, tandem learners are responsible for their own and (via the principle of reciprocity) their partner's learning.

In its original form, of course, tandem language learning is conducted face to face, which means that although learning activities may involve reading and writing, the primary channel of communication between tandem partners is oral. Whether conducted as an extension of classroom learning or as an approach to learning in its own right, a typical tandem partnership entails that the partners meet on a regular basis and divide their time equally between their two native/target languages. This in turn means that they alternate between the roles of learner and native-speaker assistant, and it is from this alternation that the peculiar power of tandem learning derives. In the role of learner, one is supported by a native speaker in one's attempts to (i) communicate in the target language and (ii) perform whatever learning tasks one has chosen; in the role of native speaker the support that one gives one's partner generates a multitude of insights into the forms not only of one's own but of one's target language, since the difficulties one's partner experiences arise partly from differences between target language and mother tongue. When pursued consistently, a tandem language learning partnership is one of the best ways of developing one's metalinguistic awareness. More generally, its interdependent processes are one of the best ways of developing the autonomy of independent learners.

Face-to-face tandem partnerships are difficult to organize on a large scale for one very obvious reason. In Manchester, for example, there are many more native speakers of English learning German than there are native speakers of German who want to improve their English; and in Bielefeld there are many more native speakers of German learning English than there are native speakers of English who want to improve their German. This practical barrier was one of the reasons why the International E-Mail Tandem Network was established by Helmut Brammerts and colleagues at the *Ruhr-Universität Bochum* (see Little and Brammerts, 1996). Increasingly universities provide their students with access to e-mail, so why not use e-mail to develop tandem language learning partnerships? Learners can register with the Tandem Dating Agency, which will assign them a partner, and the International E-Mail Tandem Network website provides them with some suggestions as regards learning activities and the management of their learning. When the Network was first established there were high hopes that tandem language learning by e-mail would bring about an international revolution in independent language learning. But this failed to happen, apparently for two reasons. First, learners did not come to the International E-Mail Tandem Network with developed skills of self-management and second, the number of people who can sustain a maximally open and individual programme of learning is very limited indeed.

Those of us who remain convinced of the special power of tandem language learning have sought to overcome this problem by embedding tandem partnerships in a tightly controlled organizational framework. For example, CLCS collaborated with the *Seminar für Sprachlehrforschung* at Bochum in a two-year project (1996–98) that linked an extra-curricular course in German for Irish students with an extra-curricular course in English for German students. The two courses followed exactly the same project-based structure (briefly referred to above), which meant that students in Dublin and Bochum were working on similar projects with similar themes at the same time. Dublin and Bochum students were paired in tandem partnerships and were expected to use their e-mail exchanges to support the development of their respective projects. Our report on this collaboration (Little *et al*, 1999) details the many practical problems that we ran into – structural differences between the Dublin and Bochum academic years; technical and organisational difficulties in collecting e-mail data; the inevitable drop-out from extra-curricular courses. One member of the CLCS team, Christine Appel, has solved the technical problem by creating a web site dedicated to tandem learning by e-mail (Appel and Mullen, 1998). This has brought both pedagogical and research benefits. Because learners visit her web site only for the purpose of language learning, their learning activity is arguably more tightly focused; also, it has been possible to devise various ways of supporting learners on-line. At the same time, all texts generated within the web site are automatically collected and may be used as research data (learners are made aware of this before they register), and Appel is currently exploring the use of computational linguistic tools to analyse her corpus.

Our experience of tandem language learning by e-mail, and in particular the need to construct adequate forms of social-interactive support, has led another member of the CLCS team, Klaus Schwienhorst, to experiment with tandem learning in the MOO. MOO denotes a text-based virtual reality in which potentially unlimited numbers of learners can communicate with one another in real time via their computer keyboards – talking by writing (for an introduction to MOOs, see Schwienhorst, 1998). Currently Schwienhorst is collaborating with a colleague in the *Fachhochschule Rhein-Sieg* on an experiment in tandem language learning using a combination of MOO and e-mail. As in our earlier experiment with Bochum, the collaboration brings together two language courses, a German course for Irish students of computer science and an English course for German students of the same subject. When differences in term/semester structure permit, the Irish and German students meet for an hour each week in the MOO, where they collaborate on bilingual learning tasks. The MOO automatically records their interactions, which they can print out for subsequent reference and analysis. Between MOO sessions, tandem partners communicate with each other by e-mail and in this way continue to support each other's project work. The combination of synchronous and asynchronous text-based communication on which this experiment is founded generates two forms of social interaction that are peculiarly apt to encourage and support individual-cognitive reflective processes – partly because they use the written channel and partly because the provision of feedback that is fundamental to tandem learning necessarily sharpens learners' metalinguistic awareness. Irish and German tandem partners communicate with one another via e-mail entirely on a self-access basis. The fact that they do so willingly seems to arise from the social relationships that they form with their partners by meeting them regularly in the MOO.

4 Conclusion

Let me conclude with a brief summary of my argument. Human learning is the product of a complex interplay between social-interactive and individual-cognitive processes. Neither of these dimensions is more important than the other, though in time and with practice we can learn to internalize (some parts of) social interaction as psychological process. According to this view of learning, learner autonomy is a matter not only of the individual's psychological relation to the process and content of learning but of his or her integration in the social-interactive practices of the learning community. This implies that independent language-learning schemes must work hard either to provide for the social-interactive dimension by other means (as in tandem language learning in the MOO) or else to engage learners in activities that help them to internalize social interaction as psychological process. Especially in the latter enterprise we shall do well to remember that proficiency in any language is founded on procedural skills, and procedural skills need exercise if they are to develop. In particular, if we want our independent language learners to become fluent in oral communication we must lay on them with the necessity to speak. If we fail to do so, we fail also to recognise a fundamental reality of language learning.

So how independent can independent language learning really be? By now it will be clear that my answer to this question is: a great deal less than is sometimes imagined, especially by university administrators intent on saving money. The practical examples I have offered in substantiation of my answer all point to one basic principle: independent language learning cannot be left to technical installations, however efficiently they may be managed. Such installations may enable us to economise in some ways, but they will never allow us to do without teachers and advisers. In universities, as elsewhere, success in independent learning will always depend on the provision of appropriate social-interactive support, and in the matter of independent language learning that means not just human beings, but highly skilled, and thus highly paid, human beings.

References

Ackermann, E. (1996) 'Perspective-taking and object construction: two keys to learning' in Kafai, Y. and Resnick M. *Constructionism in practice. Designing, thinking, and learning in a digital world*, 25–35. Mahwah, N.J.: Lawrence Erlbaum.

Appel, C. and Mullen, T. (November 1998) 'A common gateway interface for tandem language learning', paper presented at the International Congress on Technology in Teaching, jointly organized by IATEFL Computer SIG, TESOL-Spain and Universidad Europea de Madrid.

Astington, J, W. (1994) *The child's discovery of the mind.* London: Fontana Press.

Baltes, P. B. and Staudinger, U. M. (1996) 'Interactive minds in a life-span perspective: prologue' in Baltes P. B. and Staudinger U. M. *Interactive minds: life-span perspectives on the social foundation of cognition*, 1–32. Cambridge University Press.

Crystal, D. (1998) *Language play.* Penguin.

Deci, E. L. with Flaste, R. (1996) *Why we do what we do. Understanding self-motivation* New York: Penguin.

Karlsson, L, Kjisik, F. and Nordlund, J. (1997) *From here to autonomy. A Helsinki university language centre autonomous learning project.* Helsinki University Press.

Lave, J. and Wenger, E. (1991) *Situated learning: legitimate peripheral participation.* Cambridge University Press.

Lazenby Simpson, B. (1997) 'An examination of learners' preferences in self-access study and their perceived benefits for language learning' in Little, D. and Voss, B. *Language centres: planning for the new millennium*, 82–96. Plymouth: CERCLES.

Little, D. (1999) 'Developing learner autonomy in the foreign language classroom: a social-interactive view of learning and three fundamental pedagogical principles' in *Revista Canaria de Estudios Ingleses* 38: 77–88.

Little, D. and Brammerts, H. (1996) 'A guide to language learning in tandem via the Internet', *CLCS Occasional Paper* 46. Dublin: Trinity College, Centre for Language and Communication Studies.

Little, D. and Ushioda, E. (1998) *Institution-Wide Languages Programmes.* CILT in association with the Centre for Language and Communication Studies, Trinity College Dublin.

Little, D., Ushioda, E., Appel, M. C., Moran, J., O'Rourke, B. and Schwienhorst, K. (1999) 'Evaluating tandem language learning by e-mail: report on a bilateral project', *CLCS Occasional Paper* 55. Dublin: Trinity College, Centre for Language and Communication Studies.

Maturana, H. R. and Varela, F. J. (1987) *The tree of knowledge. The biological roots of human understanding.* Boston and London: Shambhala.

Nelson, K. (1989) *Narratives from the crib.* Harvard University Press.

Salomon, G. (1993) *Distributed cognitions. Psychological and educational considerations.* Cambridge University Press.

Schwienhorst, K. (1998) 'The 'third place' – virtual reality applications for second language learning' in *ReCALL* 10.1: 118–126.

Tizard, B. and Hughes, M. (1984) *Young children learning. Talking and thinking at home and at school.* Fontana.

Vygotsky, L. (1978) *Mind in society. The development of higher psychological processes.* Harvard University Press.

Vygotsky, L. (1986) *Thought and language.* MIT Press.

Wells, G. (1987) *The meaning makers. Children learning language and using language to learn.* Hodder and Stoughton.

Wenger, E. (1998) *Communities of practice.* Cambridge University Press.

Teaching culture to language undergraduates: the language issue

Nicole Mcbride ● *University of North London*

1 Introduction

In the portfolio of skills of all twenty-first century graduates, the Nuffield Languages Inquiry includes 'the ability to operate in other languages and cultures' and 'to be effective communicators' (The Nuffield Foundation, 2000: 54). The final report states that 'for many, using languages will be a regular supporting feature of their work' (ibid). This prompts a question for the language teacher: can higher education (HE) claim to be able to address this challenge if even future language graduates do not make regular use of the target language as a supporting feature of their study?

While the approach taken in secondary education has consistently referred to 'the desirability of using the target language as the "normal", "natural" or "principal" means of communication in the classroom' (Dickson, 1996: 1),[1] the situation in HE is less orthodox. The reports published by the Higher Education Funding Councils (HEFC) following the cycle of teaching quality assessments in 1995–1996 may comment on the existence or absence of language policies but they rarely make a prescriptive recommendation (see McBride, 2000). One refers to 'the issue for French providers' of 'whether to use French as the language for classroom teaching' (HEFCE, 1996a: 2) and another observes how rare it is 'to find an established policy on the use of the target language in teaching, particularly within the content curriculum' (HEFCE, 1996b: 5). Language practice in this context varies widely, from one university to another, from one language to another within the same university and even from one individual to another within the same department or school.

Decisions to use the target language (TL), English or a combination of both in the teaching of target culture[2], even when based on strong professional convictions, can lead to contradictory approaches. For example, in a context of diminishing student numbers, some departments see an increased use of the target language as a factor to attract more students to language study, others revert to English so as not to alienate them. Local and national constraints play a part in the decisions: modular frameworks make it possible to open up cultural modules to mixed language groups and to non-language specialists. Yet while this provides more viable teaching groups it results in English becoming the necessary language of delivery.

Even though the language choice may not rest entirely with the individual teacher it still is one of the key issues facing the teaching of languages in HE in the new century. This chapter investigates the language used in the teaching of cultural modules and whether established language policies are in force or decisions left to individual initiatives. It is based on the analysis of two recent surveys – a staff survey and a student survey – undertaken in language departments in UK universities between Easter 1999 and Easter 2000. These allow a comparison between practices and perceptions of teachers and the experience and expectations of students.

After introducing the two surveys and examining the cultural modules provision available to language undergraduates, the chapter will focus on the following issues and attempt, in each section, to compare teachers' and students' views:

a. Language used for the mediation of cultural knowledge (teaching and assessment).
b. Attitudes to the use of the target language in the teaching of target culture.
c. Learning components considered most important in studying culture.

2   Context: the two surveys

2.1   Teacher survey

Between mid-March and June 1999, university language departments were circulated with a questionnaire[3] via electronic discussion lists, e-mail or post. By the summer of 1999, 146 valid replies had been received from staff in language departments or schools across 77 UK universities.

Representation was well distributed:

- across the HE sector in the UK, i.e. a comparison of the actual number of universities replying with the number of HE institutions offering language degree programmes in the UK, yielded a proportion of 79%;
- across the four regions (Figure 1);[4]
- across languages: of the thirteen languages represented in the survey, French accounted for 47%, German for 22%, Spanish for 16%, Italian for 6%. The

remaining 9% included Portuguese, Russian, EFL, Dutch, Arabic, Luxemburgish, Chinese, Swedish and Welsh;
- across the different types of universities (Figure 2): this addresses the distinction between **older** and **newer** universities referred to by a number of respondents. Using Coleman's classification of universities in four groups depending on the dates when they were established (Coleman, 1994)[5] has allowed the analysis to account for the specificity of the UK provision, while preserving anonymity for individuals and universities.

England	Northern Ireland	Scotland	Wales
62/78 (79%)	2/2 (100%)	8/11 (73%)	5/6 (83%)

Figure 1: Geographical representation in the survey

University type	Proportion of universities taking part in the survey
Pre-19th century	6/6 (100%)
19th/20th century	24/28 (86%)
1960s	19/20 (95%)
1990s	28/43 (65%)
Total	77/97 (79%)

Figure 2: University sample (by university type)

The staff survey gathered information on language policies, common approaches and individual approaches. It was also concerned with attitudes and constraints both institutional and individual. Given the polarisation observed in some of the perceptions and attitudes expressed in the four university types, a complementary survey was undertaken, this time among students, to contrast teachers' perceptions with students' attitudes and expectations directly.

Detailed analysis of the staff survey is available (McBride, 2000). Some of the findings will be revisited in this article to allow comparison with the students' perceptions and attitudes.

2.2   *Student survey*

In November 1999 all the staff who had expressed a willingness to participate in a follow-up were contacted and a high proportion accepted to circulate their students with a brief questionnaire.[6] By Easter 2000, 704 questionnaires had been returned from students in 36 out of the 77 universities which had participated in the staff survey. 24% were first-year students, 31% second-year, 8% third-year (including some incoming Erasmus students) and 37% fourth-year students.

84% were native speakers of English (3% declared themselves as bilingual), other native speakers included French (4%), German (3%), Italian (2%), Spanish (2%), other European (2%) and non-European (3%).

78% were studying French, 26% German, 32% Spanish, 10% Italian and 5% another language.[7]

As can be seen in Figure 3, the distribution of staff and students returning questionnaires across the four types of universities was proportionally comparable.

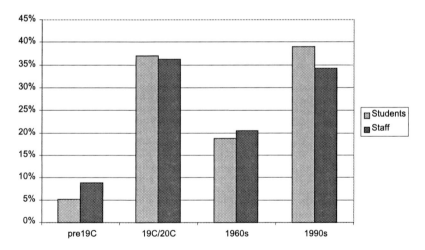

Figure 3: Sample representation across institutions

The student questionnaire concentrated on current practice experienced by students, on the students' attitude to the language used for the teaching of content/culture and on their expectations and preferences. Further sections in the questionnaire collected students' views regarding (i) curricular and extra-curricular elements considered most important in the study of culture and (ii) use of the TL for teaching by native speakers or by non-native speakers of the relevant language.

To allow comparison, some of the questions asked were common to both questionnaires.[8]

3 Cultural modules provision available to language students across the sector

The staff survey provided information on the range of subject areas available to students specialising in language in the UK. As can be seen in Figure 4[9], results pointed to strong similarities between the four types of universities. Literature was the prevailing discipline taught in 83% of the participating universities. It was listed by 92% of the staff teaching in older universities (pre-19th century and 19th/20th century), by 87% in the 1960s group but by 64% only in the 1990s group (on a par in this latter group with politics and film studies). Film studies and history came in second and third positions overall. Thus, even though literature is still the most widely available discipline in language degrees, the HE sector offers a wide diversification in its approach to culture.

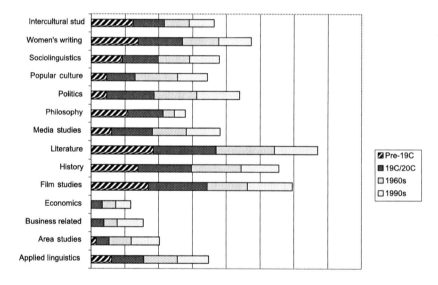

Figure 4: Provision of cultural modules

While the survey provided information on the range of courses/modules available to language students it did not yield information about which of these courses were effectively chosen by students nor about the proportion they represented within the language degrees on offer in the different universities. This aspect was not covered in the student questionnaire either. In one of the questions (question C4) students were asked to state what language they would prefer to be used in the subject areas they studied as part of their degree. They spontaneously provided the following list of subjects given below in descending order of frequency: literature, history, grammar, politics, culture, linguistics (and sociolinguistics), area study, society, European studies, economics, media studies (including cinema and television), technical modules, philosophy, translation studies, business, stylistics, law, intercultural studies, geography, art.[10]

4 Language(s) used in the teaching and assessment of cultural modules

4.1 The staff survey

41% of the respondents to the staff questionnaire reported applying departmental language policies when teaching content courses, and for a third the language used was the TL (target language). Only two of the languages overview reports produced by the Higher Education Funding Councils refer explicitly to language policies. The German report states that 'few institutions have an established policy for use of the target language; teaching entirely in German and related languages is the norm in less than twenty per cent of institutions' (HEFCE, 1996a: 9), while the report for French mentions that '30 per cent of reports draw attention to the absence of an agreed policy' (HEFCE, 1996a: 4).

In the survey comparison between the different university types showed a clear divide between the newest universities (the former polytechnics), where 60% declared a language policy' and the other three groups, where the proportion was not higher than 30%. Apart from a minority who defined their department policy as professional freedom left to individual lecturers or to the learner/teacher group, many expressed their policies in relation to levels in the students' competence and/or stages (usually years) in the degree course. Among other factors taken into account were the types of activity (teaching or assessment, and within teaching: lectures, seminars, handouts), the discipline taught and the group constituency. Overall, greater use of English was expected for assessment purposes. When variations or pragmatic constraints were not specified in the policies, respondents usually indicated that these were implemented with a degree of flexibility.

Although only 4 in 10 respondents to the staff questionnaire reported the existence of a policy, a detailed analysis of individual strategies showed that two thirds of the sample applied approaches commonly agreed within their language group or department. Overall, 42% of the lecturers used a combination of English and target language in their teaching (i.e. for lectures and seminars) of target culture, a quarter used English as the sole language of delivery and a slightly lower proportion used the target language. There again the main deciding factors quoted by staff were the students' linguistic levels and/or the stage they had reached in their degrees. Individual practices, as reported in the survey, confirmed that the target language was used even less for assessment (Figure 5).

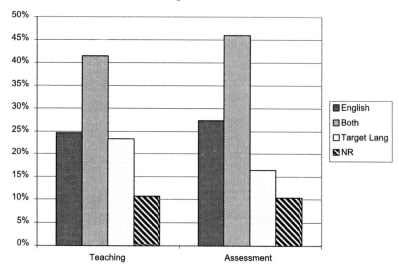

Figure 5: Individual practice in the teaching and assessment of target culture (staff survey)[11]

Considerable variation could be observed when comparing the language chosen according to university types. Figure 6 contrasts respective practices in teaching (lectures, seminars, handouts) and highlights how little use of the target language was reported by the respondents in the pre-19th century group. Further analysis showed that English was the language used by half of the lecturers for lectures and assessment, while two thirds of them described seminars as taking place in a mixture of English and the target language. In sharp contrast, over a third of the respondents in the 1990s group stated that teaching was delivered in the target language and a quarter expected the target language to be used for assessment.

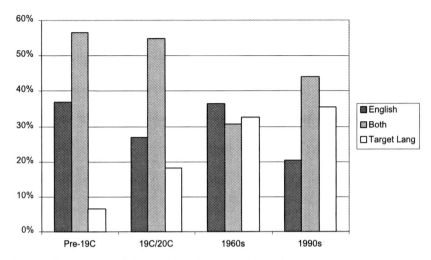

Figure 6: Language used for teaching (by university type)

4.2   The student point of view

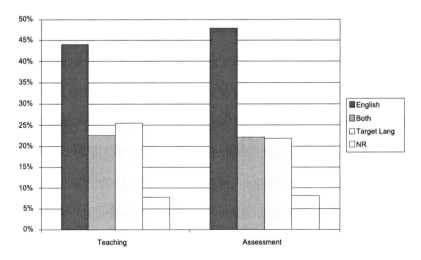

Figure 7: Individual practice in the teaching and assessment of target culture (student survey)

The results returned by the student survey, in terms of language used for the teaching and assessment of cultural modules, indicated some differences between teachers' and students' perceptions. Students reported a much higher use being made of English as the language of teaching (44%) than of the combined approach (23%) (Figure 7). Staff had a reversed perception with a much larger percentage (42%) reporting a combined approach and only 25% use of English (see Figure 5).

The same pattern of perceptions applied in the reporting of the language chosen for assessment.

When students expressed preferences there was a clear majority of them to advocate use of the language they came to study either in combination with English (45%) or as the main mediator (30%) (McBride, 2001a). These preferences were further reflected in comments spontaneously made by students across the four types of university: 'we should really experience as much as we can in the language we are learning', or 'what's the point in taking a foreign language degree' [… if the target language is not used]? The use of the target language was being seen by some as 'an opportunity to practise the language skills in an environment where they're not the main skills being assessed'. On the other hand 'less practice of French, the reason we or I am studying', as well as 'laziness, lack of exposure to the language I came to learn, lack of immersion, missed opportunity, not pushing ourselves enough, not enough of a challenge' were drawbacks commonly quoted in relation to the use of English for the mediation of content courses (for further analysis see McBride, 2001b).

5 Staff and student attitudes to the use of the target language

As well as considering classroom practices the two surveys attempted to characterise attitudes to using the target language within the context of the content curriculum. In their questionnaire, staff were presented with the following three statements and asked to choose the one with which they agreed most:

    a. You cannot teach cultural knowledge without using the target language.
    b. If you use the target language it is at the expense of depth.
    c. It is irrelevant which language is used when teaching cultural knowledge.

Responses to this question revealed an even divide among staff between statements (a) and (b) while only 14% replied that the language used was irrelevant. However, when the results are set out by university type, distinct approaches are apparent. The older the university type, the more widely shared was the belief that using the target language was at the expense of depth. This was corroborated by additional comments made by the respondents throughout the questionnaire: using the 'TL means sacrificing depth of content' (pre-19th century university); 'we do not consider that you can study the literature or history to the same depth by using the target language' (19th/20th century university). Inversely, the more recent the university type, the larger was the proportion of academics sharing the conviction that the target language was essential in the teaching of the target culture. 'Teaching in the target language may facilitate the acquisition of cultural knowledge' (1990s university); 'linguistic knowledge and contact with the target language are essential in teaching/learning cultural knowledge ...' (1960s university). As can be seen in Figure 8, the 1960s group was almost equally divided between these views. In fact, the last quotation continued as: '... but teaching in the target language does not in itself guarantee cultural learning, nor is 100% use of target language indispensable for cultural learning'.

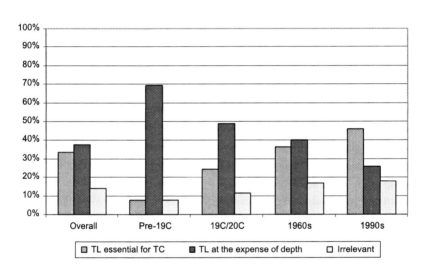

Figure 8: Attitudes of staff regarding use of target language in teaching target culture (from McBride, 2000: 33)

Comparing the attitudes expressed by staff with the language they chose for the delivery of cultural modules showed a consistent pattern: those who, in their majority, prioritised intellectual depth favoured the use of English, those who believed in the target language being essential for the teaching of target culture tended to use the target language on its own or, depending on local circumstances, in combination with English.

Students' answers to the corresponding question brought to light rather different attitudes (Figure 9). Half of them, fairly evenly distributed across the four types of university, stated that the target language was essential. Lack of depth was clearly not perceived as a main concern by the majority, though it was mentioned by over 30% of the students in the 19th/20th century group. The analysis of the student data seemed to indicate that grouping according to university types was much less significant for students than it was for staff. On the issue of language choice, students tended to share common views across the four university types.

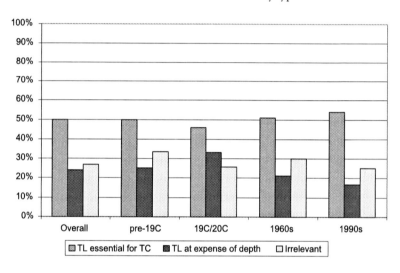

Figure 9: Attitudes of students regarding use of target language in teaching target culture

6 Components considered most important for the study of culture

Staff and student views were also compared in relation to curricular and extra-curricular aspects considered important for the mediation of cultural knowledge.

In the two questionnaires, participants were asked to assess the relative part played by four aspects of the language-learning experience: **language teaching, non-language modules** (e.g. literature, area studies), **contact with native speakers** and **placement abroad**. Ranking was by means of a five-point scale in which 1 was equal to most important.[12]

Comparison of the components given first rank by the highest number of staff and students pointed to major differences between the two groups. 40% staff placed **Cultural modules** first; over 30% chose **Language teaching** and **Placement**, and less than 10% **Contact with native speakers**. In contrast an overwhelming majority of students (65%) rated **Placement** first and over 40% chose **Contact with native speakers**. Clearly experiential learning was rated more highly than taught activities which were quoted by fewer students: less than 30% mentioned **Language teaching** and not even 20% considered **Cultural modules** as most important for 'learning about the culture of another country'. Further analysis of the data did not establish a connection between students' reactions and whether they had already completed (or were going to undertake) a mandatory placement abroad.

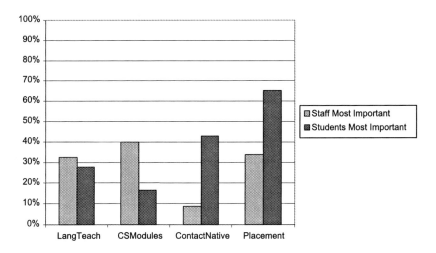

Figure 10: Perception of most important component by staff and students

7 Conclusion

While the results of the staff survey confirmed some expected general trends for the UK such as a majority using a combination of English and target language in the teaching of content course and target culture, they also revealed significant differences in the way issues were perceived and addressed in the four types of university constituting the HE sector.

Comparison of these results with those of the student survey indicated that the grouping in university types seemed less relevant for students. Students, in their majority, rated the use of the target language as essential for the teaching of target culture. Where staff were divided, students presented a more common front and the clear message emerging was a call for more exposure to the target language in its different manifestations. For example, students rated experiential learning higher than staff who tended to bring teaching activities to the forefront. In the current HE environment, where students' learning needs play an increasing part, such a disparity of views is significant. The particular emphasis laid by students on placement abroad underlines the attention to be given to the effective integration, or at least inclusion, of a placement abroad in language degree programmes. Similarly, the high rating of 'contact with native speakers' by students points to the benefits that could be reaped from imaginative curriculum developments bringing together home and foreign students taking modules in our universities.[13]

This paper has concentrated on selected aspects of the two surveys. In its detail, the staff survey points to strategies which vary to adapt both to perceived student needs and to institutional and national constraints. The student survey may provide some helpful pointers and one of them may be that, in this context also, 'English is not enough' (The Nuffield Foundation, 2000).

Notes

1   The National Curriculum (for Modern Foreign Languages), in its note about using the target language, states that 'pupils are expected to use and respond to the target language, and to use English only when necessary (for example, when discussing a grammar point or when comparing English and the target language)' (National Curriculum, 2000).

2   i.e. content or cultural courses. In the context of this research, they include those areas of the language degree curriculum, which are not primarily concerned with language teaching but with the study of Literature, Film Studies, Media Studies, History, Politics, Area Studies, Applied Linguistics.

3   The staff questionnaire has been published as one of the appendices in McBride, 2000.

4   The first figure is the number of universities replying, the second the number of potential universities offering language with cultural components.

5   Coleman distinguishes between pre-19th century universities (Oxford, Cambridge and four Scottish Universities), 19th/20th century universities (Colleges of the University of London, the University of Wales, Manchester, Birmingham, Leeds, Southampton, Bristol ...), the 1960s universities (Kent, Surrey, Ulster, Strathclyde, East Anglia, Essex, Warwick ...) and the 1990s universities (the former Polytechnics: Westminster, Portsmouth, Wolverhampton, Central Lancashire, Oxford Brookes, Caledonian ...).

6   See Appendix.

7   The total is more than 100% as some students were studying more than one language. For further detail on the profile of the survey students see McBride, 2001a.

8   Responses to the questionnaires have been analysed using specially commissioned databases (Microsoft Access) linked to Microsoft Excel and SPSS.

9   Figure 4 lists the cultural modules quoted by respondents. Results are presented as individual and cumulative percentages for the four types of institution. The horizontal axis maximum is therefore 400%.

10 For further analysis of this question, see McBride, 2001b.

11 Figure 5 includes 'no reply' (NR) returns. Slightly different percentages would have been shown if the analysis had been based solely on the replies given by respondents in this section of the questionnaire rather than on the whole survey sample (see McBride, 2000).

12 Both in the staff and in the student surveys some respondents allocated equal first ranking to two or more components.

13 Cormeraie (2000: 262–272) provides an example of a bilingual peer learning French–English module for economists, recently developed within a postgraduate course.

References

Coleman, J. A. (1994) 'Institution-Wide Languages Programmes in British higher education: National problems and perspectives' in Parker, G. and Reuben, C. (eds), *Languages for the international scientist*, 45–67. London: CILT/AFLS.

Cormeraie, S. (2000) 'Towards a language of intercultural communication: the emergent frontier space in language and cultural studies' in McBride, N. and Seago, K. (eds), *Target culture – Target language?* 252–274. London: CILT/AFLS.

Dickson, P. (1996) *Using the target language: A view from the classroom.* NFER.

Higher Education Funding Council for England, *Subject overview report 2/96. Quality Assessment of French 1995–1996* (HEFCE, 1996a), www.qaa.ac.uk/revreps/subjrev/All/qo02_96.htm

Higher Education Funding Council for England, *Subject overview report 3/96. Quality Assessment of German and related languages 1995–1996* (HEFCE, 1996b), www.qaa.ac.uk/revreps/subjrev/All/qo03_96.htm

McBride, N. (2000) 'Studying culture in language degrees in the UK: Target culture – target language? A survey' in McBride, N. and Seago, K. (eds), *Target culture – target language?* 19–80. London: CILT/AFLS.

McBride, N. 'The students' voice' in *Proceedings of the 5th annual cross-cultural capability conference, revolutions in consciousness: local identities, global concerns in languages and intercultural communication, 2–3 December 2000.* Glasgow University, 2001a.

McBride, N. 'The prime vehicle? Report on two surveys conducted in UK universities contrasting staff and student perceptions and attitudes'. Paper given at the *Globalisation, foreign languages and intercultural learning* conference organised by SIETAR, APU and South Bank University. London, 9–10 February 2001b.

The National Curriculum Online, *Modern foreign languages*, www.nc.uk.net/servlets/NCFrame?subject=MFL. HMSO, 2001.

The Nuffield Languages Inquiry, '*Languages: the next generation*'. The Nuffield Foundation, 2000.

Appendix

Student Survey

Studying culture in language degrees in the UK

> The aim of this survey is to consider existing practices with regard to the language used in the teaching of non-language modules in Language degrees. **Please, feel free to add further comments when filling in the questionnaire.**
>
> A summary of your group responses will be available to your lecturer. No individual, course or university will be identified in the publication of the overall results.
>
> *Nicole McBride, University of North London, (n.mcbride@unl.ac.uk)*

Please fill in or tick, as appropriate:

A.1. What language(s) are you studying? . . . .

A.2. What is the title of the degree you are studying for? . . . .

. . . .

A.3. In which university? . . . .

A.4. Which year of study are you currently on? . . . .

A.5. Have you completed your placement abroad?

☐ yes   ☐ no   ☐ not mandatory

A.6. What was your language level at entry on the course *(Beginner/GCSE equivalent/Post A level equivalent)*? . . . .

A.7. Your native language is: . . . .

B.1. Module/Course *(e.g. in Literature, Politics, Media studies, History, Area studies, NOT Language)* during which this questionnaire is completed:

. . . .

B.2. Which language(s) is(are) used <u>in this module</u> *(e.g. English, language of study, both languages)*

for lectures: . . . .   seminars: . . . .

handouts: . . . .   assessment: . . . .

The questions below do not refer to a specific module or unit.

C.1. Does the approach mentioned in B.2. apply to:

☐ all   ☐ most   ☐ some   ☐ none of the other non-language modules that you have taken/are taking for your degree.

C.2. If the language of teaching is not the same for all non-language modules in your course,

do you know which language will be used before you choose a module?

☐ yes   ☐ no

do students have a say in the choice of language?

☐ yes   ☐ no

does the language used depend on the stage (or year) in the course?

☐ yes   ☐ no   ☐ don't know

C.3. State your language preferences for each of the following:

	in the language of study	in English	making use of both languages
Lectures			
Seminar			
Handouts			
Assessment			

Further comments: . . . .

. . . .

C.4. In which modules do you/would you prefer:

English to be used?. . . . .

the language of study to be used? . . . .

C.5. When you started your degree did you expect all non-language modules to be taught:

☐ in English   ☐ in the language of study?   ☐ you didn't know

C.6. Does your participation depend on the language used?

☐ yes   ☐ no   ☐ not really

Do you feel you participate …

more	less	no difference	when...
			the language you are studying is used.
			English is used.
			both languages can be used.

C.7. Do you prefer lecturers to teach in their mother tongue?

☐ yes   ☐ no   ☐ don't mind

Do you find it artificial to be taught by non-native speakers in the language of study?

☐ yes   ☐ no

Comments: . . . .

C.8. In general, how would you describe your attitude to:

– being taught in the language you are studying (in non-language courses or modules)? You …

☐ prefer it ☐ resist it ☐ enjoy it ☐ resent it ☐ don't mind

– being assessed using the language you are studying? You …

☐ prefer it ☐ resist it ☐ enjoy it ☐ resent it ☐ don't mind

– participating in the language you are studying? You …

☐ prefer it ☐ resist it ☐ enjoy it ☐ resent it ☐ don't mind

D.1. In non-language courses, what advantages do you see in using English?

. . . .

What are the drawbacks? . . . .

. . . .

What advantages do you see in using the language of study?

. . . .

What are the drawbacks? . . . .

. . . .

D.2. Which do you agree <u>most</u> with?

☐ To learn about another culture it is essential to use the language of that culture.

☐ Using the foreign language is at the expense of depth.

☐ It is irrelevant which language is used to learn about another culture.

Comments: . . . .

D.3. What, in your opinion, is most important for learning about the culture of another country? *(rank from 1 'most important' to 5 'least important')*

– language teaching 1 2 3 4 5

– non-language modules *(e.g. literature, area studies)* 1 2 3 4 5

– contact with native speakers 1 2 3 4 5

– the placement abroad 1 2 3 4 5

– other *(please specify):* 1 2 3 4 5

The European Language Portfolio: a major step on the road to learner autonomy

Vicky E Davies and Michael R Jones ● University of Ulster

1 Origins of the European Language Portfolio

In 1998 the Committee of Ministers of the Council of Europe, in their *Recommendation No R (98) 6* to member states regarding modern languages, recommended that the following measure be implemented:

> *(Member States should) encourage the development and use by learners in all educational sectors of a personal document (European Language Portfolio) in which they can record their qualifications and other significant linguistic and cultural experiences in an internationally transparent manner, thus motivating learners and acknowledging their efforts to extend and diversify their language learning at all levels in a lifelong perspective.*

For the purposes of implementing this measure, the Council looked to the European Language Council (ELC) which had been launched in the previous year by a consortium of Universities throughout Europe. Thanks to the personal initiative of Dr Wolfgang Mackiewicz of the Free University in Berlin and under the umbrella of CERCLES (*Confédération Européenne des Centres de Langues de l'Enseignement Supérieur*), the ELC had come into being, with the aim of unifying and establishing standard practices to be subsequently applied throughout third level institutions in the EU, within the realms of both language learning and performance assessment (Forster Vosicki, October 2000). A number of committees were set up, each comprising an international panel of experts drawn from a range of institutions in the various states. Each committee was given a working brief to establish a code of best practice within a distinct area of language learning and teaching.

One of the objective areas was concerned with the portfolio approach within the sphere of independent or open-access learning and the establishment of mutually agreed standards which would be accepted throughout the EU as defining the level of proficiency to be achieved by any student in any particular language.

Since the ELC had drawn in many of the experts previously associated with the Council of Europe's language learning research groups, it was natural that the latter should turn to the same body to run the portfolio scheme. The ELC set up a working group (Piloting the European Language Portfolio in the higher education sector in Europe), the main end-products of which were an agreed portfolio model – the so-called Swiss version[1] – and a call to members to volunteer their particular institution to participate in the pilot run in the session 1999/2000 (Forster Vosicki, October 2000).

Fourteen institutions across Europe responded to the original call, eleven of which actually took part, including the Universities of Aston and Ulster in the UK. The management of the project was located at the Universities of Lausanne and Bremen.

The European Language Portfolio (ELP) prototype subsequently developed comprises three parts in accordance with the Common European Framework of Reference:

- a passport recording formal qualifications in an internationally transparent manner;
- a language biography describing language knowledge and learning and cultural experiences;
- a dossier in which learners' own work can be included as evidence of skills.

Its intention is that when any graduates of a European university seek employment, they would be able to present the portfolio as part of their credentials. This, like an artist or graphic designer's portfolio, would document and authenticate the level of their language abilities in any language of which they were claiming a knowledge.

The goal of the project was to create a new breed of 'linguistic freemovers' who would be totally mobile in terms of their professional and vocational lives and able to transcend national boundaries in their search for jobs, unburdened by the current impedimenta which the non-compatibility of standards in language proficiency assessment currently give rise to between the nations in Europe.

The ELP is written up by and remains the property of each individual learner and is intended to be an ongoing record of his or her language-learning experiences. It is not a snapshot of finite duration, but constitutes the documentation of an evolving organic process of language learning, which therefore has no fixed shelf-life.

2 The ELP at the University of Ulster

One of the primary reasons for the involvement of the University of Ulster was its participation in SMILE (Strategies for Managing the Independent Learning Environment), a three-year project (1997–2000) supported by the Fund for the Development of Teaching and Learning (FDTL), which sought to bridge the gap, identified in several of the overview reports on the quality assessment of modern languages (1995/96), between the provision of self-access facilities and actual student use thereof. Whilst the basic premise of the project was to encourage and promote the role of the Open Learning Adviser as the prime facilitator within the language-learning centre itself, two of its stated aims would seem to encapsulate the function of the ELP (Project SMILE,1997–2000):

- to ensure a better match between the provision of resources for modern languages and students' perceptions of their learning needs;
- to involve learners and teachers in the effective use of independent learning strategies in and out of the classroom.

It was as a direct result of the fact that the SMILE structure was in place that the University of Ulster was able to participate in the ELP project, supported by the existence of a number of internally funded projects[2] which sought to promote reflective learning within and without the classroom in both discrete and transferable modes. The goal is well-expressed by Boud (1995: 27):

> … it is fundamental to higher education that students learn to become independent of their teachers and that they should be placed in circumstances in which they are expected to make decisions about what and how they learn more often than is commonly the case at present.

The original cohort of approximately 60 language undergraduates involved in Semester 1 (October 1999–January 2000) of the pilot scheme at the University of Ulster covered not only all three year groups, but also a number of Erasmus exchange students from other European countries.

The conscious decision was taken to issue a copy of the portfolio to every student in each class targeted, as it was felt that the selective allocation thereof would have led to a wave of resentment among students not selected, and the likelihood that selected students would have seen themselves too readily in the role of guinea pigs. It was felt that such potential disaffection, whatever its roots, would necessarily have materially damaged the prospects of success of the project as a whole. Thus we accepted from the outset that the final numbers would decrease, due to the expected return of some students to their home universities after the first semester and to the disappearance of a number of students from the target teaching groups of the lecturers concerned in Semester 2 (February–May 2000). As a result, by the beginning of Semester 2 the target group had been reduced to around 40 students.

This paper therefore examines the experiences of the University of Ulster in the implementation of this instrument intended 'to allow for the recording, planning and validation of lifelong language learning inside and outside the educational context' (11 Minutes of the ELC Work Group, Jyväskylä, 1 July 1999).

In the first instance the paper looks briefly at the practicalities of implementing such a scheme from both a staff and student perspective and the effectiveness of the ELP as a recording tool in its current format, before going on to examine and evaluate its influences as we perceived them.

3 Implementation

The chosen method of evaluating the project as suggested by the Working Group was by means of a series of questionnaires to both learners and teachers at three different stages throughout the year.[3] The Ulster team chose to supplement this by collecting student statements at certain crucial points of the document and subjecting them to a close evaluation (Forster Vosicki, July 2000: 18). This method not only provided us with a wealth of factual information about what the language-learning experience of our students had been, but also enabled us to extract much useful statistical material in the process. This material was, of course, sent to the project co-ordinators to be fed into the overall assessment process undertaken on behalf of the Council of Europe.

The practicalities of implementation highlighted the, in some ways, inordinately time-consuming nature of the exercise as conceived by the pilot scheme. The latter had clearly been primarily designed to address the school situation where the teachers involved have very close and frequent contact with the pupils concerned, whose self-discipline is, to a certain extent, dictated by the learning environment. In the case of university students who, in large measure, have to discipline themselves and may see the teacher/co-ordinator only once a week, the pressure to actually return the required material according to a fairly strict timetable varied greatly according to the individual's perception of the project's intrinsic worth, and also of its relative importance in their own hierarchy of priorities. Clearly the variables are considerable at this level. The academic timetable in the UK differs considerably from that of Switzerland: no allowance was, however, made by the working group for such discrepancies. A prime example was the absolute insistence that the final returns be made in May, at what is, in the UK, the height of the examination period, a time when both the students and the staff involved clearly have other, more immediately pressing commitments.

4 Pedagogical process and progress

The stated pedagogical function of the ELP was to stimulate motivation for language learning and encourage learner autonomy and responsibility. The suggested basic premise is that, in the current higher education system of both the UK and the Republic of Ireland, curricula rarely address the broader issues of self-motivation and independent learning. In other words, we are referring to the widespread tendency to spoon-feed rather than to encourage student reflection on content and process. Thus the first major implication of the ELP was that one had to begin by explaining carefully to the student participants that it was not an examination or testing type environment that they were moving into. Instead of having their every move monitored and assessed by teachers, the latter would simply facilitate or assist them to reflect upon and to discuss with their peers the ways in which they had experienced language in the past, in both a formal and informal context, and how this had shaped their current attitude to language acquisition. Unsurprisingly, perhaps, the new scenario was one which they found very difficult to grasp. The notion that they should assess themselves largely autonomously and lay claim to specific levels of competence in various languages filled them with trepidation, and thus they required a considerable degree of nurturing before they felt able to make such self-judgements without anyone holding their hand. Kelly (1996: 94) expresses this process in the following terms:

> *Learners need to undergo a considerable transformation of their beliefs about language and their role as learner in order to be able to undertake independent learning effectively.*

The crucial factor in this process was the table of self-assessment checklists for the different languages. These finely-tuned criteria, the product of several years of consultation by European language experts within the framework of the Council of Europe, were generally very successful in enabling students to arrive at a reasonably accurate assessment of where they were at in any individual language. They ranged incrementally from absolute beginner's level to that of complete mastery of the language concerned and allowed the student to include experience not only from formal teaching and immersion visits, but also from informal contact through, *inter alia*, the compilation of a language biography. Indeed, it is our contention that the very process of writing the language biography was pivotal, not only to the evaluation of linguistic competence, but also to the triggering of the reflective learning process, which in turn led to the identification of individual learning goals.

The evaluation of the student questionnaires and of the other documents which the students produced led us to challenge a number of popularly held, yet manifestly erroneous notions concerning the hierarchical importance of the four basic language skills: reading, writing, listening and speaking. This was borne out by the high level of unprecedented student honesty and a clear reluctance to claim fluency despite the fact that many were clearly able to function at a comparatively high level in the language. This was partially to be explained by the fact that they took as a guiding principle their ability in the written mode, simply because their formal language education had taught them to believe that this skill was the more important indicator of their actual competence than, for example, oral proficiency, particularly in a functional context. Through personal reflection, students were able to identify the reasons for this differentiation in competence *vis à vis* traditionally identified language skills and also to flag up those areas where future competence would be necessary as imposed by the exigencies of real life employment. An important point is that the acquisition of language skills all round was enhanced in the minds of the students and they accorded it a much higher level of importance than previously. There was, consequently, an increase in the degree of appreciation of their own self-worth with respect to the range of skills already acquired and those to be developed by the end of their degree course and beyond.

A further outcome of the exercise was that it significantly raised student awareness of the very real practical value of even a relatively basic competence in an individual language, in terms of ensuring effective communication where otherwise none could have occurred.

With respect to the teachers, they saw their role as fostering a process of awareness raising: the students were actively encouraged to contribute to this process on a regular basis by discussing the content and issues of the ELP informally amongst themselves. In this scenario, the Learning Advisory Service afforded by the SMILE project proved invaluable, clearly mirroring Esch's (1996: 42) description of its function:

> *Its specific brief is to improve students' 'learning to learn' ability. It is a system of intervention which aims at supporting students' methodology of language learning by ... using language in the framework of social interaction to help students reflect on their learning experience, identify inconsistencies or changes and steer their own path.*

In this context, therefore, we believe that some, more insightful students have in fact progressed from a state of reflective learnership to engage in the cyclical process of the 'action researcher' (Lomax, 1995):

> *The enquiry goes beyond merely finding a technical solution to a concern, and involved the researcher in achieving a deeper understanding of the values that underpin her own and others' practice, and how these relate to the chosen outcomes.*

5 Conclusion

Essentially, the process inherent in the whole ELP project was one which looked back at past experiences in a conscious attempt to optimise its productive aspects, so as to mobilise them in a fresh context and to establish new and critical patterns of thought and behaviour which would influence and enhance future undertakings. This corresponds to Brockbank and McGill's value position (1993: 4) whereby 'people are abundant in the resources of their experience which they bring to situations that are intentionally about creating learning in learners'.

Whilst the main thrust of this reflective process is to be seen within a linguistic context in terms of this particular project, it is self-evident that such analytical reflection can be transposed to other areas of learning in two distinct ways:

• the conscious harnessing of language-learning strategies identified as a result of the ELP to other areas of learning.

• the ability to reflect on other types of learning strategies successfully employed elsewhere in the learning environment, which in turn can be applied in relevant future learning situations.

This dual capacity brought about through self-reflection bears out Shuell's contention – and more recently Biggs's model (1996, 1999) of 'constructive alignment' – that it is 'helpful to remember that what the student does is actually more important in determining what is learned than what the teacher does' (Shuell, 1986: 429). It goes without saying that the promising nature of the pilot study is a clear indicator that the working group should be encouraged in its endeavours to take this forward on a broader front as a lynchpin in the drive for learner autonomy throughout education.

It is our firm belief, therefore, that not only has the ELP experience afforded students the opportunity to reflect and consolidate their language-learning experiences hitherto, it has also equipped them with a powerful toolbox of strategies which they can use or adapt as the learning situation demands. The transferable skills element, whilst ostensibly a by-product of the ELP project, in fact supersedes the original aim in that it transcends the specific to embrace the generic and thus empowers the student for a lifetime of learning experiences.

Notes

1 For a downloadable version of the ELP visit www.unifr.ch/ids/Portfolio/#esp
2 The Tandem Learning Project (promoting cultural and linguistic enhancement through co-operative learning) and The Presentation Skills Project (integrating key skills into the curriculum using technology) funded by the Educational Development Unit, University of Ulster.
3 A full description and analysis of the questionnaires can be viewed in the final report: www.fu-berlin.de/elc/elp_pel/elp_en.doc

References

Biggs, J. B. (1996) 'Enhancing teaching through constructive alignment' in *Higher education research and development*, 12: 73–86

Biggs, J. B. (1999) *Teaching for quality learning at university*. The Society for Research into Higher Education and Open University Press.

Boud, D. (1995) *Enhancing learning through self-assessment*. Kogan Page.

Brockbank, A. and McGill, I. (1998) *Facilitating reflective learning in higher education*. The Society for Research into Higher Education and Open University Press.

Esch, E. (1996) 'Promoting learner autonomy: criteria for the selection of appropriate methods' in Pemberton, R. *et al* (eds) *Taking control: autonomy in language learning*. Hong Kong University Press.

Forster Vosicki, B. (July 2000) *Piloting the European Language Portfolio in the higher education sector: final report*. European Language Council. www.fu-berlin.de/elc/elp_pel/elp_en.doc

Forster Vosicki, B. (October 2000) 'Piloting the European Language Portfolio in the higher education sector: An ELC/CEL transnational project' in *ELC Newsletter 6*. www.fu-berlin.de/elc/Bulletin6/english/forster.html

Kelly, R. (1996) 'Language counselling for learner autonomy: the skilled helper in self-access language learning' in Pemberton, R. *et al* (eds) *Taking control: autonomy in language learning*. Hong Kong University Press.

Lomax, P (1995) 'Action research for professional practice' in *British journal of in-service education*, Vol 21: No. 1: 1–9.

Project SMILE: www.hull.ac.uk/smile/index.htm

Schuell, T. J. (1986) 'Cognitive conceptions of learning' in *Review of educational research*, 56: 411–436.

Focus research in modern languages: creating a 'powerful learning environment' for students, with students

Marina Orsini-Jones and Glynis Cousin ● Coventry University

> Child : 'Teacher, what did I learn today?'
> Surprised teacher: 'Why do you ask that?'
> Child: 'Daddy always asks me and I never know what to say.'
> (adapted from Papert, 1996: 14)

1 Introduction

The aim of this paper is to report the outcomes of a two-year investigation into language students' perceptions of their learning at Coventry University and to discuss their implications for the creation of an effective learning environment. Both authors are members of an interdisciplinary task force for teaching, learning and assessment. One (Orsini-Jones) is subject leader for Italian and teaching and learning fellow in the School of International Studies and Law and the other (Cousin) is a senior research fellow based in the Centre for Higher Education Development (CHED) and is charged with giving pedagogical research support to colleagues on the task force.

The research support provided by the CHED offered a unique opportunity to investigate students' orientation towards teaching, learning and assessment in modern languages at a time in which the sector is experiencing one of its worse crises. It was hoped that the research would throw some light on what, in the new jargon of HE, have become 'customers' attitudes and expectations' regarding their learning environment; such findings, it was felt, could inform new ways of delivering the languages curriculum at Coventry. It was also hoped that the meta-reflections about learning carried out with students would help them in the process of 'learning how to learn'.

71

As we will describe below, we conducted focus group research with students in the academic years 1998/99 and 1999/2000. We followed Krueger's (Krueger, 1994: 7) definition of focus group research, viz:

> A *focus group is a carefully planned discussion designed to obtain perceptions on a defined area of interest in a permissive, non-threatening environment. It is conducted with approximately 7 to 10 people by a skilled interviewer. The discussion is comfortable and often enjoyable for participants as they share their ideas and perceptions. Group members influence each other by responding to ideas and comments in the discussion.*

Broadly, we furthermore followed Krueger's (Krueger, 1994) methodological guidelines for gathering and analysing the students' comments. However, we have also integrated into our analysis comments received from students arising out of changes we have made as a result of the focus group feedback. The emphasis in our presentation of data and in our discussion from this research is on language-specific questions, though we think that many of them are transferable to other subject areas. Firstly, we will summarise our data (gathered both formally and informally) and secondly explore what we think they imply.

2 Research data and findings

2.1 The first set of data

This was gathered among first year students (50) during the induction week for the BA Modern Languages and Joint Degrees with a language in academic year 1998/99. Students were asked to consider the following range of questions:

1. What is learning?
2. How do I learn?
3. What do I learn fast and why?
4. What do I learn slowly and why?
5. When do I learn?
6. What environments help me learn faster?
7. What qualities do I expect from a teacher/lecturer to help me with learning new subjects?
8. How can I improve my learning techniques?

In the students' words, learning was defined as 'the acquisition of new knowledge' and also as a 'cognitive process: learning to adapt to a new environment'. They also stated that they learnt languages better via:

- constant repetition/practice;
- experience;
- fun;
- aural and oral exercises;
- help from friends who were native speakers (school exchanges were mentioned in this context).

Grammar was identified by many as a part of the learning process they did not enjoy, because they found it 'tedious'.

With reference to less language-specific, more general points about the learning process, the most common responses were:

- *Tutors should be approachable;*
- *Learning needs to be fun;*
- *Lecturers should be patient, friendly and helpful;*
- *A language needs to be practised every day, we need to be under pressure;*
- *Sometimes we need music, other times complete silence;*
- *We need encouragement, understanding, advice and honesty;*
- *We need an environment where we're involved;*
- *We need to learn with friends;*
- *The learning needs to be dynamic.*

2.2   *The second set of data*

This was gathered again in the academic year 1998/99. Self-selected groups of students were invited to lunch-time meetings – with lunch provided – in which the researcher asked questions on the students' perception of their learning environment and of the teaching. Students from all years (apart from those on placement abroad) were involved in the focus group research – ten from the first year, six from the second and eighteen from the final year. Students used this occasion to air views and anxieties in confidence as the lecturer was not present during their sessions with the group facilitator. In order to progress their feedback in ways that could be used openly and be of general use to colleagues, students were then asked to identify the attributes and qualities that make up a 'good' lecturer. The following list represents a distillation of their comments:

- **Professionalism** – references were made to respect for student confidentiality, respect for students and respect for colleagues;
- **Lecturer commitment** – students said that lecturers must have 'their hearts in their subject'; comments focused on the infectious nature of enthusiasm and of its opposite;

- **Lecturer patience** – references were made about the need for information to be repeated as often as needed; grasping a language includes a good deal of listening and memorising and students were anxious that if they did not 'get it' first time, they would not be put down;
- **Communication** – students did not want to be left struggling alone with their learning; they needed an environment in which they could openly communicate their learning difficulties;
- **Student diversity** – an appreciation of diverse cultural backgrounds and needs was seen as an important question for language learners, but this issue also concerned diversity in terms of personality and learning approaches;
- **Research** – students do not want to be subordinated to the research needs or interests of lecturers; teaching is a commitment not a duty.

2.3   *The third set of data*

The final piece of research data collected concerns a further cohort of first-year language students in academic year 1999/2000 (roughly 40) who took part in an induction week seminar and were invited to answer the question 'what really helps me to learn a language?'. Overwhelmingly, the responses to this question centred on communication and many echoed comments already reported above in indicating what was central for them:

- *Working in groups playing relevant games;*
- *Socialising with people from the country;*
- *Using the target language in the classroom;*
- *Speaking with other people;*
- *Speaking to native people;*
- *Practising the language through games and oral sessions;*
- *Speaking with friends;*
- *Being forced to communicate;*
- *Listening to others.*

3 Harnessing students' views: setting the 'ground rules'

As can be seen, some of the students' comments are fairly predictable, but in making sense of them overall, a concern for the affective side of learning comes to the fore, particularly when placed alongside some of the confidential feedback we also received. It seemed important to students to get the emotional context of learning right and this led us to create space for first-year students reading Italian in the academic year 1999/2000 (sixteen) to formulate ground rules for effective communication and learning. An 'open workshop', in which both lecturers involved in the running of the Italian core module were present, was dedicated to this aim. The researcher facilitated a discussion which included concepts of students' rights and responsibilities and those of the lecturers. The results of this discussion were agreed with students and then copied to each of them in the following form:

- *Engage with cultural differences;*
- *Create a friendly, relaxed atmosphere;*
- *Communicate in the target language;*
- *Encourage team work;*
- *The right to positive feedback;*
- *The right to speak openly;*
- *The right not to be put on the spot by lecturers or peers;*
- *The right to enjoy lessons;*
- *Encouragement of discussion;*
- *Adult to adult relationships;*
- *Patience towards learners;*
- *Tolerance towards each other;*
- *No single person to dominate discussion;*
- *No non-contributors to discussion;*
- *No expectations for too much too soon;*
- *Approachable lecturers.*

The lecturers also pointed out that in order for the above ground rules to work, the following should be agreed by students:

- *Regular attendance to language classes;*
- *Doing homework;*
- *Preparing for seminars;*
- *Coming to see lecturers during designated tutorial contact hours;*[1]
- *Respect for assessment guidelines;*
- *Punctuality;*
- *Realisation that lecturers are human beings too.*

These two lists were displayed for students to see with the understanding that any item could be re-negotiated and that others could be added. After the initial session with the students in year one, students reading Italian in year two (fifteen) were also consulted. Interestingly, they came up with ground rules similar to those which had been drawn up by their peers in the first year. The outcomes from both cohorts of students were then discussed by the researcher and the lecturers involved.

Our concern was that a thirty-minute exercise might have fading impact as the weeks progressed and we felt it important to revisit this issue at the end of the first term to check students' perceptions. In the event, students were unanimous in the view that the ground rules had been useful. Here is a selection of comments:

- *We would like the protection of agreed ground rules in every class we do;*
- *This should be a university-wide practice;*
- *The ground rules have made the atmosphere relaxed but not so relaxed that lecturers don't care what you do;*
- *Having this relaxed atmosphere means that you enjoy what you are learning;*
- *I feel under pressure in another subject where this doesn't happen, where it's not relaxed and you feel under pressure because of it;*
- *Our regular attendance on this module definitely relates to how relaxed we feel.*

We were pleasantly surprised by this feedback: it was clear that students had valued the exercise greatly. The latter proved in fact to be a 'motivator enhancer' *per se*, as students felt empowered by it. The above outcomes tie in with research about motivation in L2 learners both by Gardner (Gardner, 1985) and by Dörnyei and Csizér (Dörnyei and Csizér, 1998). According to our findings, the ten + one commandments identified by the two latter authors apply *verbatim* (see also www.linguanet.org.uk/research, Dörnyei and Csizér, 1998):

1. Set a personal example with your own behaviour.
2. Create a pleasant, relaxed atmosphere in the classroom.
3. Present the task properly.
4. Develop a good relationship with the learners.
5. Increase the learner's linguistic self-confidence.
6. Make the language classes interesting.
7. Promote learner autonomy.
8. Personalise the learning process.
9. Increase the learner's goal-orientedness.
10. Familiarise learners with the target group culture.
11. Create a cohesive learner group.

Although our research confirms the above eleven commandments, it also adds the local dimension of two extra commandments, one of a generic nature, applicable to all learning ages, and one more specific to the HE sector:

12. Be very patient.
13. Create an adult-to-adult relationship with the learners – with accommodating switches to 'nurturing parent' (Berne, 1996).

Entwistle (Entwistle, 2000) argues that encouraging students to adopt a deep, strategic approach to learning, rather than a surface, apathetic one, requires a total re-think of the student-teacher relationship. He usefully summarises the research into creating 'effective learning environments' addressing this imperative and upon which we draw for our discussion.

4 Issues for discussion

4.1 Communication and language learning

Arguably, a distinctive need among language learners centres on issues of communication. Given that getting the lines and modes of communication are a priority for any language teacher, we would argue that developing a hospitable learning environment is paramount. The evidence we collected from our focus group research and the discussions we conducted at induction sessions point to the particular usefulness of setting ground rules in this context.

4.2 The affective domain and a 'safe' learning environment

We think that the information we have collected extends the importance Krashen and Terrell (Krashen and Terrell, 1983) have placed on the affective domain in language learning. In many respects, our evidence supports their view that learning is 'affectively' filtered and that good teaching must concern itself with this. Krashen and Terrell offer insights into students' emotional readiness for language learning, suggesting that teaching should be relevant, meaningful and emotionally manageable to the student so as to lower the affective filter through which they learn: learner anxiety has to be reduced for effective learning to take place. Krashen and Terrell's remedy for this reduction tends to centre on curriculum and teaching method changes. While these changes are important, our students' feedback implies that they need to be supported by an engagement with 'safety' needs in Maslow's sense of the term (Maslow, 1987).

Our research suggests that student safety needs concern the 'learning relationship' both among peers and between students and lecturers, highlighting the relevance of Maslow's perspective on a hierarchy of human needs – in which elemental ones for shelter, food and safety need to be met before people can self-develop (Maslow, 1987). It furthermore highlights the relevance of both transactional analysis (Berne, 1996, see 4.3 below) and of Ackermann's perspective on cognitive growth as a dance between 'privacy' (stepping out) and involvement (diving in) (Ackermann, 1996).

For our students – and doubtless many others – safety issues concern the right to be respected, to be given time to think and learn (patient teaching), appropriate pace of teaching (not too much too soon), to be free of put-downs from lecturers and to learn within an environment which stimulates and supports cognitive growth both in independent settings and face-to-face with peers and tutors.

4.3   Adult to adult

An interesting side of the student feedback related to the social positioning of students in relation to lecturers. The right not to be put down, to be treated as adults, emerged in a number of the discussions in various forms. Making sense of classroom dynamics through a transactional analysis (Berne, 1996) would be of use here. According to transactional analysis, all human relations are a configuration of familial ones and each configuration structures the feelings and responses of the participants. Either we are positioned as a 'child', a 'parent' or an 'adult' with others. None of these roles are intrinsically negative because each may be appropriate at different times. For instance, a grown man playing cricket will play best if he is positioned as a 'child' because this will access his playfulness. From this perspective, adults often replicate the power relations in families at work, for instance, a style of managing that is close to the 'parent' role will invite workers to behave like 'children'. Similarly, in the classroom, lecturers who position themselves as parents will encourage their students to be dutiful sons and daughters or rebellious children, depending on the model of parenting the lecturers use. A reading of our students' comments points to a desire for a mix of adult-to-adult and parent-to-child (meant in terms of a positive nurturing role) relations to maximise learner confidence and comfort – see the thirteenth commandment above.

4.4   Diving in and stepping out

Our students' feedback confirms that 'subjectivity', 'standpoint' and 'context' (Ackermann, 1996) need to be at the centre of any discussion about knowledge and learning. Cognitive growth is not a smooth process: it results from a tension between diving into a learning environment and stepping out of it. We need to step back and think and then become immersed again: 'without connection people cannot grow, yet without separation they cannot relate' (Ackermann, 1996: 32). Ackermann also stresses the importance of accommodation: the way in which people 'loosen their boundaries' is a key element to learning. This is particularly true for language learners: 'the projections of self-in-context are a major key to learning' as they are also a key to survival in the foreign culture, language, country. Our students stressed their willingness to act out role-plays: they know that often their performance in the foreign language is proportional to their engagement with the context of the country or countries where that language is spoken and to their ability to 'become others' (Ackermann, 1996: 33). For this reason language learners reject and resent the teaching of grammar in a non-contextualised, non-relevant way. Grammar will be perceived as 'tedious' by language learners if its teaching is not customised to the students' learning needs and learning context.

5 The ICT twist: harnessing motivation via WebCT

By way of a brief aside to this research, we think it relevant to note our growing involvement in using technology to support our aims. At the time in which we were carrying out the focus group research with language students, our university introduced a campus-wide revolution in the shape of a new electronic learning environment (Orsini-Jones and Davidson, 1999) called WebCT (see Figure 1). WebCT comes with an in-built evaluation survey for each module which is electronically processed and where students can enter anonymous open-ended feedback: 'three things you like about this module', 'three things that can be improved upon'.

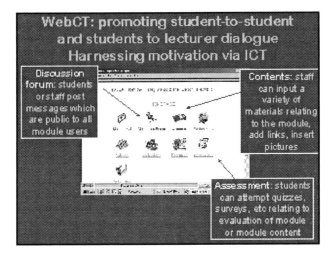

Figure 1: WebCT – an electronic learning environment

The above survey was administered on-line to fifteen students in the final year at the end of the second term. The feedback confirmed the outcomes of the focus group research, but also showed how the communication facilities within WebCT, the discussion forum in particular (where issues about the module were aired in Italian), catered for language students' needs. There were, for example, the comments for a double language module where WebCT was used for the teaching of comparative translation studies in academic years 1998/99 and 1999/2000 (Orsini-Jones, 1999):

- *WebCT has been a useful aid to the learning allowing us contact with our teacher and each other;*

- *For this module it was interesting to see the views of other students on the 'forum', something you don't usually see;*
- *WebCT is useful when you need to contact your course lecturer or other students.*

It appears that WebCT is quite appropriate for the purpose of enhancing communication channels for the following reasons (Orsini-Jones and Davidson, 1999):

- the simplicity and flexibility of its interface;
- its immediacy – the in-built discussion forum allows the students to give feedback and suggestions while the ideas are fresh;
- the dynamic environment – it empowers students and can support the creation of powerful learning environments;
- the capacity to capture the interactions and help reflection about staff–student and student-to-student communication.

In view of the positive feedback about WebCT, with particular reference to its capability to enhance communication, it was decided that in the academic year 2000/2001 the induction on learning skills and the study skills element of all main language double modules would be partly delivered face to face and partly via WebCT. The focus group research is to be carried out on-line (see Rezabek, 2000 for details of the on-line focus group) and the ground rules will be displayed to all language students and staff in the common 'course area' for modern languages available on WebCT.

6 Conclusion: a conceptual framework for the teaching and learning agenda

Overall, we have found Erik de Corte's (1995, 2000) model of a 'powerful learning environment' a useful one because it is about establishing a fertile context for learning and for student ownership of its processes. Increasingly, good teaching is being understood to be a matter of providing good learning experiences meant both at the level of quality performance activities and of a conducive learning environment (e.g. Biggs, 1999; Papert, 1996; Entwistle, 2000). We have tried to apply this understanding to the needs of language learners in the light of students' comments.

The distinctive feature of our attempt to construct a powerful learning environment lies in the collaborative ways in which we did this **with** students rather than **for** students. By consulting students firstly about their learning, then about the kind of teaching and interpersonal relations they wanted for their learning, we were able to develop pedagogic responses tailored to their feedback. As illustrated above, we shall, for example, try to make communication routes more effective and transparent for students via the use of WebCT and maximise the discussion forum facility to promote an open discussion on ground rules for all languages.

Our aim is to produce 'a classroom culture which encourages reflection on process' (De Corte, 2000) to include the many issues we have raised on the basis of student feedback. De Corte's account of the demands this places on teachers summarises well the many elements we have tried to capture in this chapter. According to De Corte, quoted in Entwistle (Entwistle, 2000: 4), constructing a powerful learning environment places:

extremely high demands on the teachers and requires drastic changes in their role and teaching practices. Instead of being the main, if not the only source of information ... the teacher becomes a 'privileged' member of the knowledge building community, who creates an intellectually stimulating climate, models learning and problem-solving activities, asks provoking questions, provides support to learners though coaching and guidance, and fosters students' agency over, and responsibility for, their own learning.

Good learning and good teaching need to be underpinned by effective communication and an understanding that cognition and emotion are intertwined. Our findings clearly point to the need to create powerful collaborative learning environments for language learning in which students' needs are voiced and understood.

Notes

1   While an open-door policy used to exist a few years ago, the increase in the amount of administrative, teaching and research duties have made it necessary to restrict contact hours outside the classroom and to encourage students to adhere to them and/or make separate appointments via e-mail if they find the tutorial hours (called 'surgery hours' in our institution) problematic.

References

Ackermann, E. (1996) 'Perspective-taking and object construction: two keys to learning' in Kafai, Y. and Resnick, M. *Constructionism in practice:* 25–35. Mahwah, New Jersey: Lawrence Erlbaum Associates.

Berne, E (1996) *Games people play.* Ballentine Books.

Biggs, J. (1999) *Teaching for quality learning at university.* Open University Press.

De Corte, E. (1995) 'Fostering cognitive growth: a perspective from research on mathematics', *Educational psychologist,* 30: 37–46.

De Corte, E. 'Marrying theory building and the improvement of school practice' in *Learning and instruction* (in press)

Dörnyei, Z. and Csizér, K. (1998) 'Ten Commandments for motivating language learners: results of an empirical study', *Language teaching research,* 2: 203–229.

Entwistle, N. (2000) 'Constructive alignment to improve the quality of learning in higher education'. Paper presented at the Dutch Educational Research Conference, University of Leiden.

Gardner, R. C. (1985) *Social psychology and second language learning: the role of attitudes and motivation.* Edward Arnold.

Krashen, S. and Terrell, T. D. (1983) *The natural approach: language acquisition in the classroom.* Pergamon Press.

Krueger, A. R. (1994) *Focus groups: a practical guide for applied research.* Sage.

Maslow, A. (1987) *Motivation and personality.* Harper and Row, third edition.

Orsini-Jones, M. (1999) 'Implementing institutional change for languages: on-line collaborative learning environments at Coventry University', *ReCALL,* Vol 11, 2: 67–84.

Orsini-Jones, M. and Davidson, A. (1999) 'From reflective learners to reflective lecturers via WebCT', *Active learning,* 10: 33–38.

Papert, S. (1996) 'A word for learning', in Kafai, Y. and Resnick, M. *Constructionism in practice:* 9–24. Mahwah, New Jersey: Lawrence Erlbaum Associates.

Rezabek, P. (2000) 'Online focus groups: electronic discussions for research' in *Forum for qualitative social research,* 1: 1.

www.linguanet.org.uk/research, site with various articles on motivation in language learning.

http://home.edu.coventry.ac.uk/ched, site with information about focus group research and WebCT implementation at Coventry University

The quantity and quality of corrective feedback on a tandem learning module

John Morley and Sandra Truscott ● *University of Manchester*

This study set out to assess the quantity and quality of corrective feedback generated in a tandem learning scheme for undergraduate students at a British university. A further aim of this work is to develop a set of guidelines on corrective feedback for students on tandem learning schemes.

1 Introduction

Tandem learning is now being offered by many educational institutions, both in Britain and in Europe, to students who wish to learn and further develop a foreign language. It is essentially a reciprocal learning activity in which native speakers of two different languages work together, in pairs, to develop their language skills and learn more about each other's country and culture. Both partners in a tandem pair alternate between practising their target language and acting as expert sources on their own language and culture. Although a range of modes of reciprocal learning are available, including e-mail partnerships, learning in tandem often involves pairs of learners meeting regularly to collaborate on a scheme of work, which may or may not be linked to a formal course or to a system of accreditation (Calvert, 1999).

In addition to the extensive contact time with native speakers of the target languages and the possibilities for learning and practice that this provides, tandem learning in a face-to-face mode offers a number of important advantages over more traditional classroom-based learning, including:

- opportunities for students to develop learner autonomy and independence, that is, to learn to manage and direct their own learning;
- greater potential to meet specific areas of student need and/or interest;

- opportunities for learners to gain insights into the language-learning difficulties of their partners and develop a better understanding of the contrasting linguistic features of the two languages;
- less learner anxiety than is usually associated with the teacher-dominated classroom environment;
- opportunities for students to gain experience as learner mentors.

Another advantage of this kind of learning, and which is the focus of this paper, is the potential for the generation of significant amounts of corrective feedback relating to a participant's written and oral performance in the target language.

At Manchester, the tandem programme is structured around a series of collaborative learning tasks and may be followed on a one- or two-semester basis. A maximum number of 50 students are accepted. None of these students are majoring in a modern foreign language but all have attained a post-A level or equivalent standard in the tandem target language. The students are asked to work through a series of learning tasks which lead towards the compilation of a dossier. The work is credit rated at ten credits per semester. All the tasks necessitate a preparation, production and feedback stage.

The success of the project depends on the mutual support of the paired partners. It is made clear at the outset that students must be prepared to do as much for their partner as they expect their partner to do for them. This requires that they not only spend an equivalent amount of time practising each language, but that each student devote as much time to preparation and feedback as their partner. Before students meet, they prepare the topic in hand independently. Production may consist of a discussion, semi-structured interview or a descriptive monologue in the target language. During the feedback stage, students suggest where their partners could usefully improve their target language in the areas of pronunciation, grammar, lexis.

In evaluations of an earlier pilot project, students seemed generally satisfied with the corrective feedback that they were receiving. Nevertheless, there were a small number of comments relating to 'confusing feedback', 'lack of grammar explanation', and 'insufficient feedback' which we found disturbing. A review of the literature revealed that very little had been written on the kind of corrective feedback that occurs in reciprocal language learning – as we shall see, most of the research on corrective feedback is concerned with that given by teachers to students. We, therefore, set out to learn more about what was happening in the feedback stages and to try to assess the quantity and quality of corrective feedback that was being given. A further aim of this work was to develop a set of guidelines on corrective feedback that students could use when preparing and giving corrective feedback to their partners.

2 The role of corrective feedback in language learning

Attitudes to corrective feedback have altered over the years. The 1980s were characterised by a debate on the usefulness of explicit formal instruction. The usefulness of corrective feedback, considered as a form of explicit teaching, was questioned by those who subscribed to the universal acquisition theory. Supported by studies of learners' interlanguage which was characterised by a marked persistence of errors even though explicit instruction had taken place, researchers claimed that teaching could not alter the order of natural acquisition of items in the target language (Dulay, Burt and Krashen, 1982). These claims were also backed up by evidence from the experiences of children learning L1, who seemed to learn language successfully despite receiving limited amounts of negative evidence. Other arguments against error correction were associated with Krashen's affective filter hypothesis and hinged on the fact that correction might heighten a learner's level of anxiety, in turn raising the affective filter, and in so doing, impeding learning (Krashen and Terrell, 1983).

More recently, however, the role of explicit formal instruction, including the role of corrective feedback, has been reassessed. The general view now seems to be that comprehensible input, whilst necessary, is by itself not a sufficient condition for acquisition to take place. Schmidt (1992) claims that a degree of awareness is important for new material to be incorporated into the developing language system and that learning cannot take place without what he calls 'noticing'. And as a corollary, others have gone on to claim that formal instruction can facilitate the intake of unknown features of L2 by causing noticing to occur. Corrective feedback is now recognised as having a role to play, not only in facilitating the noticing of features of L2 but of learners' interlanguage errors as well. Pica (2000), for example, argues that feedback has an important role in modifying output. She writes that students 'need feedback on their production so that they can modify it toward greater comprehensibility, appropriateness, and accuracy' (Pica, 2000: 8). This is particularly important 'she adds' for more advanced students who 'seldom receive feedback on their lexical and morphological imprecisions, as long as they communicate their message meaning'.

Empirical evidence in support of these claims, however, has proved difficult to demonstrate. Nevertheless, a number of studies have shown that corrective feedback can help improve learners' accuracy under certain conditions. Carroll, Swain and Roberge (1992), for example, were able to demonstrate that corrective feedback helped adult subjects distinguish French nouns which ended in -*age* from those ending in -*ment*. In another study, Carroll and Swain (1993) investigated the different types of feedback on the learning of the dative alteration rule in English. In tests, all experimental groups that received feedback out-performed those that did not, with the groups who received overt metalinguistic feedback performing best. More recently, Doughty and Varela (1998) report a study in which a teacher gave feedback to ESL school students on past tense errors in the context of content-based teaching involving oral and written science laboratory reports. The feedback took the form of drawing learners' attention to their errors and recasting them in correct sentences that the learners were asked to repeat. After six weeks, the students who were subject to corrective feedback demonstrated significant gains in accuracy in comparison with the control groups. However, in this case, it is not clear whether the feedback that the students received or the opportunity they were given to practise repeating the correct form affected the change. One suspects, though, that both of these processes played a part.

Perhaps another reason for reassessing the role of corrective feedback is that several studies have shown that learners show a strong preference for it either from their teachers or from their native-speaker friends (see Chaudron, 1988). This would seem to undermine the objection to corrective feedback which claims that it results in high levels of anxiety. One might equally argue that not giving learners, particularly adult learners, any feedback is equally likely to raise their 'affective filters' or at any rate produce a certain degree of demotivation, disappointment or anxiety, since learners are not getting what they want and feel they need.

Other researchers have concerned themselves more with which kinds of corrective feedback are most effective. Lyster and Ranta (1997) looked at different types of corrective feedback given by teachers and noted that recasts were the most common – recasts being defined as a rephrasing of the original incorrect utterance – but that recasts were less effective in leading to self-correction than were other types of feedback. They argue that while recast may offer valuable negative evidence, students are less likely to attend to the error through self-repair. In fact, in their study, students took relatively little notice of the teachers' recasts or repeated inaccurately. Other forms of feedback, they argue, particularly elicitation, would seem to be much more effective in pushing learners to attend to, and therefore 'notice', errors in their own interlanguage.

A similar analysis of feedback type was undertaken in the current study, but in this case the corrective feedback was given by students rather than teachers.

3 Method

All students who were registered on the tandem programme were asked to record their performance on at least one task, as well as the feedback that they received from their partner for this. It was explained that the feedback element of these recordings would not be assessed, but that it would be used for research purposes. In the end, 40 recordings were selected for analysis on the basis of recording quality. This gave us eleven hours' worth of analysable material.

The production – as opposed to the feedback – component of the recordings was analysed for number of errors and for error type. For the purposes of this research, errors were defined as linguistic items which are not grammatically, semantically or phonologically well formed and which 'lend themselves to correction' by a well-educated native speaker, with an understanding of languages/language learning. Categories for coding errors were similar to those used by Lyster and Ranta (1997), that is, grammar, lexis and phonology. In this study, the grammar category included morphological forms and structural items. The lexical category included frequent word combinations (collocations) and fixed phrases, as well as single lexical items. Errors in content were not included in the analysis even though feedback may have been given for this. A number of phrase units were analysed as exhibiting more than one error type.

For the analysis of the corrective feedback a modified version of the typology developed by Lyster and Ranta (1997) was utilised:

1. **Explicit correction** is used to refer to moves in which the partner indicates an error and then provides the correct form. In our analysis this move also encompassed metalinguistic explanations; in other words, the explanation could include some grammatical metalanguage which referred to the nature of the error;

2. **Recasts** refers to simple correct reformulations of errors without explicit indications that the errors have occurred. They are not, for example, introduced by phrases such as 'you mean ...' and 'you should say ...';

3. **Elicitation** refers to feedback moves in which the student tries to elicit the correct form from their partner. In this study, elicitation principally involved asking students to reformulate an incorrect utterance;

4. **Clarification requests** are indications that the listener has misunderstood and that a reformulation is required. This was perhaps the most difficult category to record because, although many requests involve phrases such as 'I don't know what you mean by X', some may involve paralinguistic clues such as frowning or looks of puzzlement and these could not be captured in our study;

5. **Repetition** refers to feedback in which the 'correcting' student repeats the error in isolation. No other clues are given other than perhaps a slight rise in intonation.

The errors and the corrective feedback were analysed both during the tasks and after the tasks. The post-task feedback sessions on the recordings ranged in length from 2 to 11 minutes, with an average post-task feedback time of around 3.5 minutes.

4 Results and discussion

4.1 *Encouraging amounts*

Figure 1 shows the total number of error items that we detected in the production stages of the tasks according to type (n.637), grammatical errors being the most frequent category. Just under half of all the errors identified (44%) were corrected in some way by the partners, either as during-task interventions or as post-task feedback. Interestingly, the proportion of items corrected is not much below the proportion found in Lyster and Ranta's study in which teachers corrected 62% of their students' errors. It should be noted, however, that in this regard direct comparison of error treatment is problematic since Lyster and Ranta were analysing teachers' error-correction moves during communicative interactions in classrooms, whereas in the current study corrective feedback was analysed as both during-task and post-task feedback between individual learners. Nevertheless, we felt that the percentage of errors corrected by our students was encouraging.

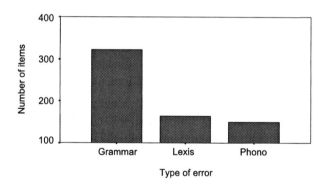

Figure 1: Total number of errors by type

The actual number and type of items corrected during task performance by the students is shown in Figure 2. The figure shows that during the tasks most of the feedback was concerned with errors in lexis and pronunciation. This is perhaps understandable since during-task feedback has to be quick and simple if it is not to disrupt task fluency, and it may be that grammatical errors are more difficult to deal with in this way since they usually require a degree of explanation. It may also be that errors in pronunciation and lexis have a greater adverse effect on the communicative quality of the interaction and as a result attract more attention. Once again we were encouraged by these results since they suggest that the students were sensitive to the need to correct where necessary, but they also suggest that the students were careful not to give feedback that might disrupt the communicative flow.

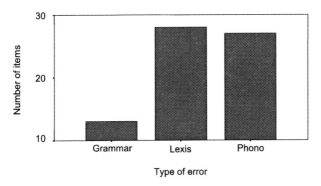

Figure 2: During-task corrections by type

4.2   Feedback as recasts

Figure 3 shows **how** students correct during the tasks. As might be expected, this feedback tends towards **recast**, the quickest and least disruptive of all feedback types.

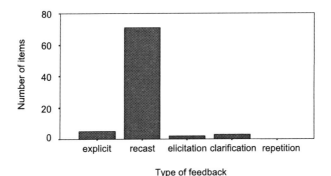

Figure 3: During-task feedback by type

Most students were able to repeat the recast in what Lyster and Ranta call 'learner uptake' – that is, some form of reaction of the student to the correction – usually in the form of 'student-generated repair'. Our findings were somewhat at odds with those of Lyster and Ranta's study which found that recasts tended to be ineffective at eliciting student-generated repair; students seemed to take little notice of the teachers' recast or repeated inaccurately. In fact only 13% of recasts in the earlier study led to repair. In our study, however, where corrective feedback was given in the form of recast, levels of uptake in which the corrected language was either repeated or reincorporated into the discourse in some way were high (around 90%). It is not clear why there should be such a difference of repair rates between the two studies. One possible explanation is that, in our study, much of the during-task feedback related to the correct pronunciation or correct choice of words in the partner's discourse, and these tended to be language items that needed to be used more than once; much of the feedback seemed to be necessary or important for our students to achieve their communicative goals. It is not clear that this was the case in Lyster and Ranta's study. The general maturity and enthusiasm of our students may have been another factor.

As a result of low rates of uptake in the classroom setting, Lyster and Ranta suggest that teachers/tutors should not rely so extensively on recasts in their correction techniques, but rather should endeavour to use techniques which encourage students to 'draw on their own resources' (Lyster and Ranta, 1997: 57). Interestingly, however, more recently the value of recast as a form of correction has been reassessed. According to Doughty and Williams, 'uptake may not be the most revealing indication of acquisition, a process that is not usually instantaneous' (Doughty and Williams, 1998: 208). In other words, even if recasts do not lead to immediate uptake, it is difficult to know what is happening long-term. Further, Doughty and Varela (1998) point out that evidence from first-language acquisition shows that parents make frequent and systematic use of recasts when correcting their children's ill-formed utterances. It might be, therefore, that students in mentor role adopted recast quite naturally as an almost incidental strategy for giving corrective feedback – and that this type of feedback is both instinctive and effective.

4.3   Post-task feedback

The number and type of correction items in the post-task feedback is displayed in Figure 4. The post-task feedback comprised approximately 75% of all the corrective feedback that was given. This in itself was encouraging since it shows that whilst some feedback was given during the tasks, most of the corrective feedback was noted down by students during the tasks for correction and possibly for discussion later, thus limiting the amount of potentially disruptive interventions. The figure below also reveals that the amount of feedback for a particular category of error was in very similar proportion to the total number of errors for each category (see Fig.1). In other words, students were not disproportionately focussing only on one or two kinds of error.

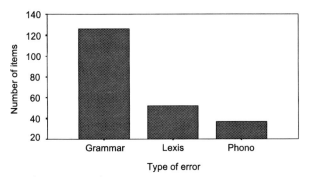

Figure 4: Post-task corrections by type

Figure 5 shows that post-task feedback tended towards the explicit. Grammar, phraseology, poor pronunciation were all brought to the attention of the students' partners, in utterances such as 'You said that, but you should have said this …'. This provided opportunities in the session for metalinguistic discussions on similar or related grammar points. The quantitative data also tells us that during post-task feedback students were not over-correcting each other; in other words, too much corrective feedback was not being given. In fact, the average number of post-task feedback items per student per task was around six, ranging from three to fourteen items. In a preliminary meeting, we had already advised students about this, suggesting that they should focus the post-task feedback on a short list of salient errors, or at any rate what they perceived to be errors (malformed utterances caused by their partner's lack of linguistic knowledge/awareness) as opposed to slips, rather than very long lists of incorrect formulations.

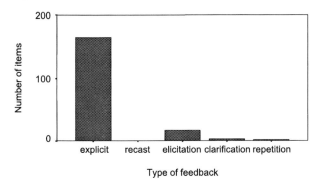

Figure 5: Post-task feedback by type

One thing that did emerge, however, upon closer examination of the corrective-feedback moves, was that declarative knowledge of formal grammar tended to be much higher in the case of the European students who, on occasions, confused home students by use of unfamiliar metalinguistic terminology. Conversely, home students confused their European counterparts by partial or even inaccurate accounts of English grammar. An example of this is seen in the exchange between a French and a British student below. In this case, the British student fails to illustrate the differences in meaning and use between 'publicity' and 'advert', revealing her confusion over the word class/noun class of the word *publicity* in the process.

A: I think you meant 'adverts'…didn't you? 'Publicity' is …

… You can't use *publicity* you know like *an advert is a publicity*. It's not a noun.

B: So when do you use *publicity* for?

A: It's like a … *a campaign*, I think. You know it's a *publicity campaign*. Things like that.

B: So … 'advert'.

A: Yeah.

It is for these reasons that we will now advise students (see Appendix) to eschew detailed descriptive treatment of grammar points and to provide instead concrete examples for the partner to come to his or her own conclusions of how the structure works. This can then be checked against the description in one of the recommended grammar books or dictionaries, or through a web-based discussion group for further comment from tutors and students.

4.4 Teacher-like techniques

Figure 5 also shows us that a number of corrective moves in the post-task feedback were categorised as elicitation. This technique takes different forms but essentially consists in mentor or teacher teasing out the correct utterance without producing it herself. This technique was used relatively infrequently by students in our group, although it did occur very successfully in at least two pairs. Elicitation, of course, is a teaching technique and our students, although cast in the teacher's role, are **not** teachers. In fact, it might be precisely because elicitation is a teacher-like technique that student mentors avoid it. They, after all, have to combat on two fronts – that of teacher and student – and moving too far into teacher terrain might compromise the student-to-student relationship. Nevertheless, Lyster and Ranta's study demonstrates that elicitation leads to a higher percentage of uptake and repair than other corrective mechanisms (Lyster and Ranta, 1997: 55), though, as we have said earlier, whether this is effective long-term is another question. In any case, elicitation would be a useful addition to our students' arsenal of strategies, even if only to add variety to the feedback session and to ensure that both participants are fully engaged.

Other types of corrective feedback, clarification and repetition, were not utilised to any significant extent by our students. There were exceptions, however. Clarification was used for asking for further explanation of content during the tasks – but very rarely for language correction – and in post-task feedback repetition sometimes tended to be combined with elicitation as a student was asked to correct his or her earlier utterance. Certainly, during the tasks, such interventions, except where understanding was at stake, might have been seen as disruptive, and both during and post task, these might also have been perceived as too teacher-like.

Perhaps the most notable variation in the quality of the post-task feedback was the extent to which students discussed the feedback. In some partnerships there was very little discussion; correct forms were simply explained or elicited before moving on. Other partnerships, however, went beyond this and engaged in contrastive analysis between target language and mother tongue or made generalisations about forms and patterns. Others combined this with contextualisation and exemplification of new or corrected language. A good example of contrastive analysis is the following excerpt from a French/British partnership. We have selected this extract because it highlights not only contrastive analysis, but also contextualisation, the giving of concrete examples, involvement with the partner and sensitivity to slips.

A: Later on, when we were doing it before, we were talking about the ages. If er … ermm … someone's … I've lost my train of thought … If someone such as … If you had children when they were quite old there'd be a big age difference between you and your children.

There's actually an expression 'age difference'. I think you said 'difference of age' or something which makes sense …

B: Yeah, because it's the word in French.

A: It's *différence d'âge*. But, erm, 'age difference' is just a way of saying it.

B: So in a sentence how could you use that?

A: 'There's a big age difference between …'

B: 'My parents and I'?

A: Yeah, you'd normally … it's often used when you're talking about, um, maybe a younger girl going out with an older man. You'd say 'Oh, that's bad 'coz there's such a big age difference.'

B: Okay, okay.

A: Yeah? And the last thing you said 'family as we knew him' and you just meant 'as we know it' coz 'the family' … You know that, don't you?

What we termed generalisation – or moving from the particular to the general – seemed to be a little more widespread than either contrastive analysis or contextualisation. As might be expected, this tended to take place in the area of pronunciation, as the problem tends to be more clearly defined. Nevertheless, there were other instances. One student, for example, gave a proficient run through of Spanish nouns with unexpected genders. Another generalised about the 'ed' endings in past tenses and how they should be pronounced.

4.5   Out-performing teachers

There were areas where we felt that students were equally good, or even outperformed teachers, not perhaps in direct relationship to error correction, but in the relationship which they formed with their partner and the atmosphere which was created within the learning session. Students, for instance, were remarkably sensitive to slips or mistakes rather than errors. (See an example of this in the extract above.) This behaviour might be due to a factor touched on earlier – students do not wish to compromise their relationship. Noticing slips rather than errors constructs rather than destroys solidarity.

Another area where student partnerships scored over conventional classrooms was the overwhelming use of the target language in the tandem session, and this applied to the giving and discussion of corrective feedback as well as to other interactive moves. Those of us who are practising modern language teachers will be well aware of the constant lapse into L1 once students are left alone to work in pairs. From the evidence of our recordings, this seldom happens in tandem programmes. Students genuinely seem to have accepted the need for reciprocity, emphasised at the outset. Similarly, students were much more proactive in tandem than in the conventional classroom. They did not simply wait to be corrected, but many spontaneously asked for further information about constructions, lexis, contextual information and so on.

Finally, and probably most important of all, we were struck by the enthusiasm and encouragement generated in some of the tandem pairs. These pairs were able to give feedback as part of a communicative rather than an isolated activity. They seemed genuinely interested in what the partner had to say and not merely how they said it and this generated discussion, questions and comments throughout. Before giving feedback, many students made observations about progress made earlier. And the feedback itself was couched in terms that could only motivate.

5 Conclusion

In this small-scale study we set out to learn more about the corrective feedback that was given by learners to their partners on an assessed mutual learning scheme. The investigation showed that whilst there was variation in the quality of the feedback that was given, and whilst attempts to draw on metalinguistic terminology to explain errors in some cases caused confusion, in general, participants received appropriate amounts of useful, encouraging and relevant feedback. Of course, we cannot be sure that the standard of feedback seen here was maintained on the unrecorded tasks which students had to complete for their tandem work. Student evaluations at the end of the scheme, however, seemed to suggest that it was, with only a few exceptions. In fact, a number of students remarked on just how valuable the feedback aspect of the work had been.

We also have seen that some of the better feedback was given using techniques such as elicitation, contrastive analysis, contextualisation and generalisation and we will want to encourage future cohorts of tandem students to make more use of these in future years. As part of this improvement, we have devised an error correction guide, which, along with a workshop on error correction, will be used with students in the next academic year (see Appendix).

References

Calvert, M. (1999) 'Tandem: a vehicle for language and intercultural learning' in *Language learning journal*, 19: 56–69.

Carroll, S. Swain, M. and Roberge, Y. (1992) 'The role of feedback in adult second language acquisition: error correction and morphological generalisations' in *Applied psycholinguistics* 13: 173–98.

Carroll, S. and Swain, M. (1993) 'Explicit and implicit negative feedback: an empirical study of the learning of linguistic generalisations in *Studies in second language acquisition* 15: 357–66.

Chaudron, C. (1988) *Second language classrooms: research on teaching and learning.* Cambridge: Cambridge University Press.

Doughty, C. and Varela, E. (1998) 'Communicative focus on form' in Doughty, C. and Williams, J. (eds) *Focus on form in the classroom: second language acquisition.* Cambridge: Cambridge University Press.

Doughty, C. and Williams, J. (1998) 'Pedagogical choices in focus on form' in Doughty, C. and Williams, J. (eds) *Focus on form in the classroom: second language acquisition.* Cambridge: Cambridge University Press.

Dulay, H., Burt, M. and Krashen, S. (1982) *Language two*. Rowley, MA: Newbury House.

Krashen, S. and Terrel, T. (1983) *The natural approach*. New York: Pergamon.

Lyster, R. and Ranta, L. (1997) 'Corrective feedback and learner uptake' in *Studies in second language acquisition*, 19: 37–66.

Pica, T. (2000) 'Tradition and transition in English language teaching methodology' in *System* Vol 28(1): 1–17.

Schmidt, R. (1992) 'Psychological mechanisms underlying second language fluency' in *Studies in second language acquisition*, Vol 14(4): 357–85.

Appendix

Some guidance on error correction (post-task oral feedback)

1. Do not choose to correct too many errors at one session – so far, six or seven has been the average. Twelve is the absolute maximum.

2. Choose errors which are 'pervasive', 'systematic' and known to be 'remediable' (Long, 1991, 1996):

   - 'Pervasive' and 'systematic' imply that your partner has a consistent difficulty with a particular area (of pronunciation, grammar, lexis);
   - 'Remediable' suggests that correction will help your partner improve that particular point. For example, if your partner is incapable of pronouncing a French 'r' correctly, do not insist – choose another area to correct which he or she can improve.

3. Correct errors that have 'highly stigmatising effects on the listener or reader' (Hendrickson, 1978), that is, errors which might have negative practical consequences (slang, swear words).

4. Do not be afraid to correct the same error in subsequent sessions. Learners do not incorporate the right form simply because their attention is drawn to it once. Give plenty of concrete examples of errors. Try to avoid general remarks like 'you are still having problems with the past tense' – specific instances are much more helpful.

5. One useful way to correct is by repeating the sentence which contains the error, highlighting (by stress) where the mistake occurs. If your partner cannot correct him or herself, 'recast', that is, give the correct version of the original sentence and get your partner to repeat.

6. Correct one error at a time – try not to overload your partner with too much feedback.

7. Try to compare patterns and usage in the mother tongue and target language. This is called 'contrastive analysis'.

8. When correcting phonological errors, give your partner the opportunity to repeat and practise the correct pronunciation.

9. **During-task feedback**: only correct errors which are causing communication breakdown and/or are simply and expeditiously corrected.

10. Try to make the feedback session as interactive as possible. Both partners should be involved in the correction process.

Some guidance on error correction (written work)

1. We suggest that you underline mistakes such as mis-spellings, punctuation, accents and agreements. Your partner should be able to correct these him or herself.

2. Write in the correct words and phrases (recasts) as clearly as you can. (Remember that writing styles differ from one language to another and can be difficult to interpret.)

3. You could develop your own system of symbols for indicating errors and error type (e.g. @ for agreement).

4. We suggest that you try to ensure that each partner reads out loud the corrected version of the written work. (Some students have made mistakes in transferring corrections from the draft to the final copy.)

N.B. – *marks will be deducted where there is evidence of insufficient, inadequate or unhelpful feedback.*

Collaboration and the role of learner strategies in promoting second language acquisition in tandem learning partnerships

Lesley Walker ● *Modern Languages Teaching Centre, University of Sheffield*

1 Introduction

Language learning in tandem takes place when native speakers of two different languages work together in order to learn each other's language and develop a knowledge of the target culture and community. Tandem learning is underpinned by principles of **reciprocity** – both partners should benefit equally from the exchange – and **autonomy** – each partner is responsible for their own language learning, establishing learning goals and deciding on methods and materials. The data for this paper is taken from tandem learner diaries. Entries in the diary can be made in either the student's mother tongue or the target language. The diaries are those of students on the face-to-face tandem module, an assessed module run by the Modern Languages Teaching Centre (MLTC) at the University of Sheffield. Prerequisites for the module are a good A level qualification for British students and the baccalaureat for their French partners.

The examples given here are taken from 50 learner diaries.

2 Introspection and the use of learner diaries

The use of introspective techniques and the data gathered from learner diaries is open to criticism for several reasons. One might well fear, like Seliger (1983), that retrospection might lead to a more polished version of events rather than a reflective account of what actually took place. Together with Seliger, we might also fear that the data-gatherer, in this case the tandem tutor, is being humoured or given what the writer thinks she wants to read. However, retrospection has at least the advantage of taking place after the event, unlike think-aloud techniques. Here, many like

Vygotsky, quoted by Goss *et al* (1994), would argue that effective simultaneous reporting of strategy use is distorted because of the difficulty of functioning at cognitive and metacognitive levels at the same time.

Then too, the perusal of diary entries for insight into the learner's learning skills and strategy use might be self-defeating. According to Cohen (1983), it is possible that the ability to successfully analyse, reflect on and report the learning process is another aspect of the capacity for successful language learning. However, we might agree with Grotjahn (1987) and cautiously accept that such introspective data as the diary entries is at least important for framing hypotheses which could be tested later. A more positive attitude to such data is voiced by Gillette (1987) who regards the material as qualitative, revealing aspects of language learning previously inaccessible to investigation.

The problem with this sort of data is that usually we can not be sure how objective or truthful the writer is. There is no convergence of evidence. However, with the tandem learner diaries we have a very particular instance where two learners, who are working as a pair, both record the process. Each is, of course, writing from their individual point of view, but each also on occasion records the dynamics of their partnership. We have instances of the very convergence of evidence which is missing from a solely individual account. On this basis we can perhaps suspend our misgivings as to the validity of the diary entries in general.

2.1 Convergent evidence from tandem learner diaries

Partners' logging of the same circumstance in the learning process can range over many different categories, with both linguistic and affective or social content. For example, one pair write of the opportunity given to a French student to come to the English partner's party for both social and linguistic reasons.

> E1: *My partner's English has clearly improved, both in accuracy and fluency. He demonstrated this at a party at my house where, despite his being the only French speaker, he made plenty of contribution to conversation.*
> F1: *Mon partenaire m'a aussi invité à son anniversaire, où j'étais le seul francophone. Cela m'a permis (entre autres activités) de tester mes capacités avec des anglophones qui n'étaient habitués ni à ma prononciation, ni à me parler lentement. L'expérience m'a satisfait.'[1]*

Another pair provides proof of an amusing exchange of cultural knowledge to further their language learning.

F2: *Today my partner explained to me the rules of snooker. It turned out that these rules are quite complicated. The main goal is to **pot** first all the red balls but trying to pot the black ball between two successives (sic) red balls. Then you pot the remaining balls respecting the given order.*

E2: *Aujourd'hui il a voulu que j'explique les règles de snooker, parce qu'il regardait les matchs de snooker à la télé pour le championnat du monde et il ne comprendait (sic) pas les règles. Nous avons rit (sic) beaucoup aujourd'hui. Ce n'est pas étonnant qu'il le trouve très difficile parce qu'il regarde une télé en noir et blanc. Alors nous nous sommes bien amusés, qui est très important pour apprendre la langue'.*[2]

The following cultural exchange takes place at the beginning of a different tandem partnership.

E3: *We discussed how French and Brits have a need for a different amount of personel (sic) space.*

F3: *British people like a lot of space around them. They tend not to make physical contact of any kind with strangers and feel very uncomfortable if any one stands too close to them. They will instinctively draw away if anyone comes too close.*

The next pair made one of their goals helping each other to improve intonation.

E4: *Pour un accent français, c'est important de mettre l'insistance (sic) sur le dernier (sic) partie d'un mot.*

F4: *Je viens de faire prendre conscience à A que s'il voulait paraître Français, il devait placer l'accent tonique sur la finale, non sur la première.*[3]

There are many instances of partners noting the same vocabulary during the same session. A visit to the dentist prompts the following entries.

E3: la carie: *tooth decay* le dentier: *false teeth*

F3: carie: *cavity* dentier: *false teeth, denches (sic)*

Partners also note new idioms …

E5: J'ai **la** mémoire comme **une** passoire. *I've got a memory like a sieve.*

F5: J'ai **la** mémoire comme **une** passoire. *I've got a memory like a sieve./* 'siːv/

… and are delighted when they have proof of aiding the other's learning.

F6: *I am happy to hear S making progress too. It is a real pleasure to see that she remembers things I have taught her. For instance, last time, she said 'revenons à nos moutons', an idiom we had studied together.*

If we look at the partner's diary page where the theme of the session was idioms, we find:

E6: revenons à nos moutons: *let's get back to work.*

The following entries in the diaries of two partners are illuminating.

F3: Ayant remarqué qu'on utilise souvent *'get'* dans des expressions j'aimerais avoir plus de précisions'[4]

E3: *He brought an exercise on using the word 'get' with him which I helped him with.*

In addition to a vocabulary list of expressions with 'get', F3 writes,

I fully achieved today's goal, there's no getting away from it.

There is also corroborative evidence of correction

F7: *I've just realised that A. says very often 'c'est bon' instead of 'c'est bien' and before I never thought of correcting her. I need to be more rigorous.*

E7: *L. pointed out that I tend to say 'c'est bon' when I actually mean 'c'est bien'. I hadn't really noticed this and I think I do it mostly out of habit so will have to try really hard to avoid doing it in future.*

and advice on methods for learning …

E3: *I encouraged him to write down all new vocabulary in his diary.*

F3: Il m'a aidé à compléter mon vocabulaire.[5]

The extracts furnish evidence in areas we will be looking at in this paper to analyse the collaboration and the use of learner strategies to promote second language acquisition in the tandem partnership.

3   Learner strategies

In this paper the learner strategies described are the learning strategies defined by Oxford (1990). Strategies are defined as **direct** or **indirect**. Direct strategies, whose main categories are Memory, Cognitive and Compensation, are used by the learner to directly handle and process the material they are working with. The indirect strategies – Metacognitive, Affective and Social – are used at one remove to organise the learning and promote the best conditions for language learning, both personal and societal/environmental. The dual aims of the tandem learning module are to promote oral proficiency and to develop autonomy in those learners involved in a tandem partnership. It will be seen that the whole range of direct and indirect learning strategies are used by our learners and described in their diaries. At advice sessions the aim is to raise student awareness of those strategies most useful in directing their own learning. The diary pages too are designed to further learning and subsequent reflection (see Appendix). The first pages are given over to needs analysis and goal-setting tables. On the diary pages proper there are headings and spaces for goals set and new language acquisitions. On the other side of the page, the student has the opportunity to decide whether the goal was achieved, what is the next step, and can jot down anything he or she observed about their own or their partner's way of learning. Students are advised to plan ahead, to use materials and methods conducive to achieving the goal set and to consolidate any new learning. The aim is for the student to develop or acquire the metacognitive or organising skills which support effective language learning. Advice and awareness raising is also provided on the direct skills with which a successful learner manipulates language. So far there have been no explicit classes where learning strategies are taught, but a session on how to fill in the diary is provided.

4 Strategy use by the tandem pair

4.1 Goal setting and error correction

Successful strategy use by individuals is commonplace, but it is all the more striking when the range of strategies are used and their usage planned by a tandem pair. For example it is very common for students to write in their diaries, as does this student:

> E8: *During the first session I explained my long and short term goals to my partner.*

However, some students involve their partner even at this stage:

> E9: *The second step in the analysis process was to ask my tandem partner what weaknesses he could see. The response I got was that I consistently made mistakes in pronouncing certain sounds. I feel that pronunciation is hard to analyse yourself, so I asked him to specify some key sounds and working on these was my second long-term goal.*

By involving her partner in the basic need analysis and goal-setting procedures, this student has the benefit of the input of her native speaker partner. Other learners go further.

> *E5: We were both very keen to sit down together in our first meeting in order to analyse and define our specific needs. This was not only important to the way in which we were going to structure our learning together but it also gave us the opportunity to discover the level of the other's language.*

Her partner writes:

> *F5: We set our topics and goals together from the beginning.*

The use of such mutual planning strategies and supportive input can only benefit the pair. Successful learners recognise the debt to their partner, who knows what goal they are trying to achieve and helps them towards it.

> *E10: She knew I wanted to work on the subjunctive, so with lots of things I said she made me say it again in a way which required it, which was really helpful.*

Another student writes:

> *E11: We have a good relationship whereby she corrects me and if she knows there is an area I want to improve (like negative sentences for example) she'll point them out to me when she uses them and she makes more effort to correct mine.*

The area of error correction is one which is obviously very important and one in which partners again provide mutual support and advice.

When partners know each other's specific long- and short-term goals, it follows naturally that error correction feeds into working towards the goal.

> *E11: She was really helpful by always asking what my goal for the session was and interrupting to test me on it. I tried to do the same for her because it seems like a very good idea.*

The social strategies involved in error correction include asking for correction and co-operating with peers and proficient users of the target language. Error correction is an important part of the learning process and is accepted by the partners as a natural adjunct of the tandem relationship.

> *E12: Still making some lazy slips in conversation like using* envers *instead of* environ *but my partner lets me know when I do it.*

Most error correction is explicit but there are also examples of successful implicit correction.

E13: *Instead of correcting me, my partner used what I should have said in her reply or next sentence which helped me to understand the use and fix the pattern in my memory.*

Many Erasmus students understand the unique benefits of error correction that the tandem partnership affords.

F8: *She corrects me each time I make a mistake, which is really helpful, because when I talk with someone else they understand me and my mistakes and I don't know if what I say is correct or not, therefore I can't really improve.*

And English students too:

E4: *Living in France for a year … I found people are often reluctant to correct. With my partner I did not have this problem, in fact, with our intensive 'zero tolerance' correction, I soon discovered exactly where I was making the same mistakes.*

Mutual error correction is a given in tandem partnerships, forming part of the reciprocity on which each is based.

F8: *We are both trying to correct our partner as much as possible and not just trying to understand him, because it is not worth doing that.*

Of course error correction brings problems:

F6: *I don't correct her all the time because I understand what she says. On one hand it is not so good because she will do the same mistake again if I don't correct it but on the other hand it is really annoying to be stopped when you're talking especially when it often happens.*

However, partners find their own way around this obstacle

F9: *What was pleasant it's that she didn't cut me short. She always waits for me to finish with my ideas and then explains to me what was wrong.*

Others write of trying out an intensive five-minute correction session. Others evolve a system of monitoring from error correction with the mutual use of the metacognitive strategy of evaluating and monitoring progress.

E14: *As agreed at the beginning of the semester we corrected each other at the end of the session which worked well. We also took five minutes at the beginning of the session to recap on last week's work. He tested me on the expressions I had decided to concentrate on and I remembered them without any problems.*

We can see in the next entry that another pair takes error correction and the subsequent monitoring of progress one step further.

> E5: *My partner and I took pleasure and pride in re-using the vocabulary learnt in the previous sessions. Our boasting quickly became a new way of learning. If we happened to ask twice for the same word, we undoubtedly let the other know about it, and we did remember then! Just because we had been 'told off', and it was always nice and fun because of the relationship between us.*

4.2 The use of affective strategies to enhance the learning process

The string of strategies used in the game just described includes the cognitive strategy of re-use of words learned, with the accompanying memory strategy of reviewing. More importantly we notice the affective and social strategies of risk-taking in 'boasting', and 'telling off' but also empathising with others. The fact that the learning was fun brings in the affective strategy of using laughter to lower anxiety. An important element of tandem learning is the fact that it entails learning in a relaxed atmosphere with a peer. Many, many entries talk of the comfortable atmosphere and the encouragement given which helps the learning process. Graham (1997) reviewing the literature on 'interpersonal' aspects of language learning, sums up the situation. For many years it has been recognised that speaking and listening are the greatest source of anxiety among students. This problem is exacerbated, especially for girls, in a classroom situation with the teacher. The real or imagined evaluation of their peers and a fear of negative evaluation by the expert can lead to 'communication apprehension'. Tandem learning does away with this threatening environment. Both partners are experts in their own language, which builds self-esteem and leads to equality with one's learning partner. As one partner writes:

> Ce statut d'égalité met à l'aise et facilite l'apprentissage.[6]

4.3 Analysis of collaborative learning strategies

The experience of learning with a peer, and of studying what one has chosen, also feeds into an already positive learning environment. The additional element of mutual strategy use, together with the active support of one's partner, makes a unique learning situation for the benefit of both learners. The most common strategies – memory, cognitive, and compensation strategies – used by the tandem pairs are shown in Figure 1. This table shows mutual strategy use. In some cases the strategy was introduced to one partner by the other, but in other cases the strategy has been devised by the pair to suit their unique working partnership.

Strategy	Category	Mutually devised	Transferred
writing down new words	Cognitive		✓
Pronunciation practice	Cognitive	✓	✓
use of phonetics	Cognitive/Memory		✓
re-use	Cognitive/Memory	✓	✓
decision not to use dictionary but to paraphrase	Cognitive	✓	
listening for gist	Compensation		✓
guessing	Compensation	✓	
use of synonyms	Compensation	✓	
put new word in context	Memory	✓	

Figure 1: Mutual strategy use

Among the features likely to favour successful second-language development, Ellis (1985) lists:

- A high quantity of input directed at the learner;
- The learner's perceived need to communicate in the L2;
- Independent control of the propositional content by the learner (e.g. control over topic choice);
- Adherence to the 'here-and-now' principle, at least initially;
- The performance of a range of speech acts by both native speaker/teacher and the learner (i.e. the learner needs the opportunity to listen to and to produce language used to perform different language functions);
- Exposure to a high quantity of directives;
- Exposure to a high quantity of extending utterances (e.g. requests for clarification and confirmation, paraphrases and expansions);
- Opportunities for uninhibited practice (which may provide opportunities to experiment using 'new' forms).

Tandem learning provides the environment envisaged by Ellis. In addition, it takes language learning out of the traditional classroom with its inhibiting factors and provides the chance to work with a native speaker who will correct errors.

Furthermore, the effective use of learner strategies by the pair can only enhance the conditions for learning success. Ellis goes on to state that while there are strong theoretical grounds for believing that a learning setting rich in these features will lead to successful second-language acquisition, there is little empirical proof. The evidence from the diaries may be viewed as such proof.

4.4   Case Studies

Let us look at two partnerships in depth to provide us with supporting evidence that tandem learning, with its opportunities for mutual support and strategy use, promotes second language acquisition.

Partnership A

Both partners set their goals and tell their partner what they are hoping to achieve. The French partner writes:

> F10: *Pour moi le plus important était d'améliorer ma prononciation … Le travail autour de notre prononciation s'est avéré un peu plus difficile. Je me suis concentré sur le 'ough' Ma partenaire m'a préparé de nombreux exercices et m'a fait lire des articles de magazines afin de me corriger. J'ai fait la même chose pour elle car elle avait des difficultés pour différencier les 'ou' et les 'u'. Nous nous sommes beaucoup investies pour essayer d'apporter à l'autre ce qu'elle attendait de nous.*[7]

Her English partner mirrors this:

> E15: *We made up difficult sentences for each other to say in order to distinguish between sounds. For example I composed sentences involving the 'ough' sound to show the different pronunciations. She helped me to differentiate between the sounds 'ou' and 'u'.*

Here is an extract from the diary of French speaker F10, an exercise hand written by her English partner:

1. *I thought that I would sort out the papers.*
2. *I taught him how to catch.*
3. *He caught the ball which his daughter threw to him.*
4. *He fought against the illness.*
5. *She bought a can.*

It can be seen from the composition and order of the sentences how she has tried to help her partner to memorise the sounds.

Here is an extract from the diary of English speaker E15, a similar exercise in the handwriting of her French partner:

1. *Il est sous le coussin du sofa.*
2. *Ne touche pas le four car il est chaud.*
3. *Le pauvre poussin souffre de la solitude.*

Both partners write, not only of their satisfaction with their own progress in pronunciation, but also of their partner's improvement and of the pleasure they have taken in their contributive role.

Partnership B

The diary entries of this pair give us an insight into the method they evolved together which, once developed, was used successfully throughout their partnership.

The French partner describes it:

> F11: *La méthode qui m'a paru la plus efficace, c'est celle que nous avons utilisée à maintes reprises – lire le texte*

- *premier objectif, améliorer ma prononciation*
- *deuxième objectif, comprendre le vocabulaire, utiliser d'autre vocabulaire, d'autres expressions*
- *troisième objectif, résumer l'article, discuter dessus. Mon partenaire notait mes fautes lorsque je m'exprimais, ensuite nous prenions le temps de corriger toutes ces fautes, et je m'appliquais à les réutiliser correctement.*
- *quatrième objectif, la semaine d'après lorsque mon partenaire m'interrogeait, être capable de redire ce que j'avais appris sans faute et là c'était un succès.*[8]

There is evidence of this method throughout the diaries of both partners. For example, an extract from the diary of the English partner reads:

E16: Text on 'Employment' from 'The European' newspaper.

> *My partner read the text in English and I attempted to translate simultaneously. As we went through the text, we explained the more difficult vocabulary and ideas using both languages to ensure we both understood them properly. We found it became increasingly easy to change between the two languages and this helps with confidence in speaking. We both gave each other a lot of useful economic vocabulary as well as learning more about sentence structure in each language ... translation of the article enabled me to practise maintaining a good accent. I used several subjunctive constructions.*

Vocabulary entries for this session include:

F11: Do workers have the bottle (le courage) *to ride jobs slump?*

E16: to have the bottle to do something: avoir le courage de faire qch.

When the English student writes 'I feel I have achieved all of the goals I set', he echoes his partner's sentiments.

5 Conclusion

Many scholars and researchers have written about the advantages of collaborative learning. Schinke-Llano (1995) writes of the significance of Vygotskian thought to the second language acquisition process and, quoting Vygotsky, describes the zone of proximal development (ZPD) which is

> *the distance between the actual developmental level as determined through problem solving and the level of potential development as determined through problem solving under adult guidance or in collaboration with peers.* (Vygotsky, 1978, 86).

Schinke-Llano (1995) describes the desirability of activity in which two interlocutors engage in meaningful communication, the purpose of which is to move the interlocutor of lesser ability to a higher level in the ZPD through mediation from the more skilled interlocutor. Many tandem learners with the help of their partners perform beyond their competence, whether by 'closing the gap' or by learning by explaining. Psychologists, like Wood *et al* (Wood, Bruner and Ross, 1976) wrote of the 'scaffolding' process involved in helping someone to learn. A successful tandem partnership provides evidence for both theories. We may perhaps move towards a new definition of scaffolding as a proactive partnership between peers, where mutual affective and linguistic support, by means of effective learner strategies, is in evidence. Language learning is seen to flourish in such an environment, moving learning methodology forward for the new millennium.

Notes

1 The extracts given are from the diaries of English and French students on the face-to-face tandem learning module at the MLTC. E denotes an extract from an English student's diary and F from a French student's. The numbers show the different students involved.

Translation: My partner also invited me to his birthday party, where I was the only French speaker. This gave me the opportunity (amongst other things) to test my language skills with English speakers who were not used to either my pronunciation or to talking to me slowly. I was pleased with the experience.

2   Translation: Today he wanted me to explain the rules of snooker because he was watching the snooker matches on TV for the World Championship and he didn't understand the rules. We laughed a lot today. It's not surprising he finds it difficult to understand the rules because he's watching a black and white TV. So we enjoyed ourselves, which is very important in learning a language.

3   Translation: E4: 'For a French accent it's important to put the [stress] on the last part of a word'.

F4: I've just made A realise that if he wants to appear French, he has to place the stress on the final and not the first syllable.

4   Translation: I've noticed that people often use 'get' in expressions, so I'd like to have further information on this.

5   Translation: He helped me to write up my vocabulary.

6   Translation: This feeling of equal status puts you at ease and makes learning easier.

7   Translation: For me the most important thing was to improve my pronunciation. Working on our pronunciation turned out to be a little more difficult. I concentrated on 'ough'. My partner prepared lots of exercises for me and made me read magazine articles [aloud] in order to correct me. I did the same for her as she had difficulty in distinguishing between the sounds 'ou' and 'u'. We put in a lot of effort to try to provide what we expected from each other.

8   Translation: The method I found most effective was one we used on several occasions: read the text;

• 1st objective: improve my pronunciation;

• 2nd objective: understand the vocabulary, use other vocabulary, other expressions;

• 3rd objective: summarise the article, discuss it. My partner took a note of my mistakes while I spoke. Then we used the time to correct all these mistakes and I tried to reuse the correct versions;

• 4th objective: the following week, when my partner questioned me; to be able to say what I had learned without any mistakes and I was successful.

References

Cohen, A. D. (1983), 'Studying second-language learning strategies: How do we get the information?' in *Applied linguistics*, 5: 101–12.

Ellis, R. (1985) '*Understanding second language acquisition*': 161. OUP.

Gillette, B. 'Two successful language learners: an introspective approach': 269 *'Introspection in second language research'* Faerch, C. and Kasper, G. (eds)

Goss, N., Ying-Hua, Z., and Lantolf, J. (1994) 'Two heads may be better than one: mental activity in second-language grammaticality judgements': 265 in *Research methodology in second-language acquisition* Tarone, E., Gass, S. and Cohen, A. (eds)

Graham, S. (1997) *Effective language learning*: 94. Multilingual Matters Ltd.

Grotjahn, R. (1987) 'On the methodological basis of introspective methods': 70, *Introspection in second language research* Faerch, C. and Kasper, G. (eds)

Oxford, R. L. (1990) *Language learning strategies: what every teacher should know*: 17–21. Heinle & Heinle.

Schinke-Llano, L. (1995) 'Reenvisioning the Second Language Classroom: A Vygotskian Approach' in Eckman, F. et al (eds) *Second language acquisition theory and pedagogy* Lawrence Erlbaum Associates.

Seliger, H. W. (1983) 'The language learner as linguist: of metaphors and realities' in *Applied linguistics*, 4: 179–91.

Vygotsky, L. (1978) *Mind in society: The development of higher psychological processes.* Cole, M. et al (eds) Harvard University Press.

Wood, D. Bruner, J. S. and Ross, G. (1976) 'The role of tutoring in problem solving' in *Journal of child psychology and psychiatry and allied disciplines*, 17: 2: 89–100.

Appendix

Learner Diary:

Sheet 1

Date: . . . .

Today's Goal . . . .

. . . .

Topic: . . . .

<u>Vocabulary and new expressions</u>

<u>Cultural Information</u>

<u>Sentence Structures/Accuracy</u>

(Overleaf)

Did I fully achieve today's goal or not?
Yes Give evidence of achievement of goal/progress towards goal
No Give reasons for not doing so

e.g. What did I learn? Was it enjoyable, useful, interesting?
What worked/didn't work? Why? What will I change?
Am I pleased with my contribution/my partner's contribution today?
Did I receive enough help? Did I ask for help?

. . . .

. . . .

. . . .

. . . .

. . . .

. . . .

Next step

Observation of self and partner

e.g. Am I copying partner's use of grammatical structures correctly?
Am I modelling my pronunciation on my partner's?
Am I reusing the new vocabulary/structures I have acquired?

. . . .

. . . .

. . . .

. . . .

. . . .

. . . .

. . . .

Studying Russian language at university: do beginners do better?

Sarah Hudspith ⦿ University of Leeds

1 Introduction

1.1 Background

In Britain there are approximately 34 higher education establishments which teach Russian as a main subject to honours degree level.[1] The vast majority of these universities admit entrants to a programme that divides the students into two streams for language classes according to prior knowledge. Language courses are in most cases streamed for at least the first year, in many cases for two years, and merged at the latest for the final year, after a third year spent abroad with some or all of this time in Russia. Related studies offered in the degree programmes, such as literature and history, tend not to be streamed and are specifically designed so as not to favour one language stream over another. Very often, the larger of the two streams is the *ab initio* stream, while the stream for those students with A level Russian or equivalent, frequently numbers just a few. Most universities aim to bring beginners to a parity of proficiency with those students who entered with A level by the final year. Such an aim may not always be stated explicitly in university literature, but it may be inferred from the aim, held by all universities which offer both *ab initio* and post-A level Russian, to teach Russian to degree standard from either starting point.

1.2 The problem

This study raises the question of whether there is indeed a parity of proficiency by final degree level between students who enter with different levels of experience of Russian, or whether there is any evidence to suggest that one cohort performs better than another. In an education system based on equality of opportunity, it is to be hoped that where curricula are designed to this end, no one group of university entrants has an advantage over another by the time they graduate. The most recent Higher Education Funding Council for England (HEFCE) Subject Overview Report on Quality Assessment of Russian and Eastern European Languages and Studies (1996) focuses on whether institutions ensure that the *ab initio* students are not disadvantaged. It states:

> … *on nearly all programmes beginner entrants do at least as well as those with GCE A level Russian, and in some cases perform to a higher level of attainment.*

This is of course highly commendable, and universities are to be praised for the success of intensive programmes designed to achieve degree level in as little as four years. However, it is possible to view the HEFCE statement from another angle: are institutions doing as much to challenge and develop the language skills of the latter group whilst they are apart? Behind the achievement of *ab initio* students out-performing those with A level Russian, lies the possibility that those with an initial language advantage end up slightly disadvantaged. The years that the two cohorts are taught apart are crucial.

1.3   What the study covers

This study is based on the results of research undertaken in 1997/98 as assessed project work for the University of Sheffield's Postgraduate Certificate in Higher Education, with additional data from the University of Nottingham, where I was recently employed. I look first at the broad picture in England's HE institutions offering Russian. I then focus on the University of Sheffield's Department of Russian and Slavonic Studies as a case study. This university was chosen because its maximum Teaching Quality Assessment (TQA) rating of 24 suggests no obvious room for improvement within the terms of the aims and objectives that it set for itself. I present both statistical and anecdotal evidence: the former consists of TQA reports, a survey of language learning in the UK, course evaluation questionnaires (CEQs) and final degree classifications. Whilst a general trend emerges from the findings, and various reasons are offered for this trend, no conclusions are drawn due to limitations of the evidence. However, it is hoped that this study will raise awareness of the existence of a potential problem, and it identifies a subject worthy of further research.

2 The national picture

2.1   The merits of streaming

The first point which needs to be made, although perhaps an obvious one, is that there is no question that students of Russian would be better served by tuition which put beginners and students with A level together for language classes. It is clear that in order to meet the needs of such heterogeneous groups of students, separate tuition must be provided up to an appropriate level. To teach them together would overwhelm the beginners, bore the non-beginners and likely demotivate both students and staff, thus frustrating the learning process. Research has shown that whilst there are long-established convincing arguments against streaming in primary and secondary education, at tertiary level where appropriate it is pedagogically sound (Jones, Harris and Putt, 1990). The question here, therefore, is not whether streaming is appropriate but whether a necessary system is meeting the needs of all the students.

2.2   The findings: the TQA reports

Out of 27 institutions of higher education assessed for teaching quality in Russian in England in the session 1995/96, fourteen were assessed solely for Russian and Eastern European studies and languages, and the remainder were assessed for modern languages, in which the above was included (HEFCE, 1996). Out of the total, only three institutions were commended for the parity of achievement between post-A level students and *ab initio* students, which is remarkable considering that such parity is an implicit if not explicit aim of all the institutions. Some of the reports seemed to show evidence either way: one commented first that both cohorts were equally challenged and motivated, but then that the first class degrees had recently been attained only by *ab initio* students; two others remarked on parity of achievement by the final year despite various problems at earlier levels. From this evidence a picture emerges that where problems exist, they occur in the first two years where streaming is in place for at least a year.

2.3   The findings: the languages survey

Between 1993 and 1995, the European Language Proficiency Survey, headed by James Coleman of the University of Portsmouth, was conducted to investigate among other things the proficiency, progress and motivations of almost twenty thousand university students of French, German, Spanish and Russian in the British Isles. Of this number, 550 studied Russian at eleven institutions around the country.

The survey combined the use of a C-Test (Grotjahn, 1996), to measure proficiency, with an extensive questionnaire. A C-Test is a comparative test of proficiency designed for students of all abilities, with scores based upon a normal distribution. The level was set so that a score of over 25% in the first year of university for a non-native speaker was seen as a positive achievement (Coleman, 1996). Therefore, the same C-Test was given to students at all levels of their degree programme, with the exception of first year *ab initio* students, who would be expected to score zero. Coleman's findings are interesting but not wholly conclusive. In personal communication, Coleman has elaborated on the general results of his survey in order to examine the relative performances of students who studied Russian at school and students who began at university. He found that students who were in their fourth year of university and who had been studying Russian for more than four years gave a slightly higher average C-Test score than final-year students who counted four years of Russian tuition (see Figure 1).

Years of tuition	more than 4	4
Mean C-Test score (+/- SD)	50.13 (15.71)	45.16 (SD not available)
Median score	47	46
No. of students	47	61

Figure 1: Proficiency test results for final year students of Russian

Coleman suggests that the reason for the mismatch between the mean and the median C-Test scores for students who started Russian before university is that the mean may have been pulled up by a few high scorers with possible family links to the language.

In personal communication, Coleman then went on to compare the mean scores for all the number of years of past study (see Figure 2). These results show a general trend towards higher C-Test scores with increasing years of study, but within that trend there is a steady progression in proficiency for the first four years of study followed by a slight decline for the next three years of study. However, standard deviations are not known, and the small difference between the mean scores may imply that between years two and seven, the progress made is small. But in Coleman's opinion, which I share, the figures may be interpreted to suggest that proficiency in learning Russian does not increase in direct proportion to the time spent learning the language. In fact there would seem to be a slight regression for a few years before substantial progress is made. This view is supported by research, which has indicated that there is no exact correspondence between the number of years of study and levels of proficiency in listening, speaking, reading and writing:

Thompson (1996) noted that individuals who had studied Russian for the same length of time had different levels of ability, whereas other students who had studied for different lengths of time had similar skills. Of course it must be noted that Coleman's survey is a cross-sectional study which tested students of different years at the same time; there are numerous variables to take into account with a cross-sectional study, such as the possibility of a 'weak year', changes in syllabus or teaching staff and so on. However, the survey is informed by a longitudinal pilot study which tends to confirm these results, as Coleman explains:

Coleman (1996a) reports of three longitudinal studies of student proficiency within the context of the European Language Proficiency Survey. One found that, on average, a student makes nearly as many percentage points progress during two years of sixth-form study at school, as during the entire university degree course, emphasising how hard it is to make continued and even progress at advanced levels, and explaining in part the sense of frustration to which students often testify in their early years of university study. (Coleman, 1996)

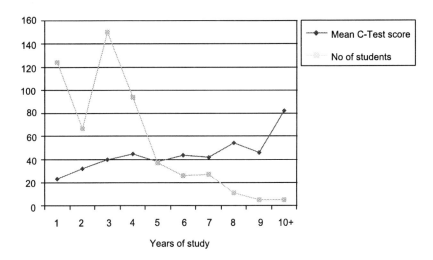

Figure 2: Proficiency test results for students of varying years of study of Russian

3 A case study of a British university

The Department of Russian and Slavonic Studies at the University of Sheffield has been chosen as a case study in order to illustrate in more detail the broad issues presented in the present study. Most interestingly, the department's maximum TQA result of 24 raises the question of whether there is any noticeable trend in student performance in a department where the assessors made no suggestions for improvement. Indeed, the TQA report praised the department for the parity of achievement between the two cohorts, but at the same time acknowledged that in the two most recent years, the *ab initio* students had done slightly better than the post-A level students, although there were 'only marginal differences between performance of the two entry streams' (HEFCE, 1996). What evidence then, may be obtained from such a department?

3.1   The evidence from students

The first place to look is clearly the degree results. The figures below from 1993 to 1997 are from Sheffield, but more recent figures were obtained from the Department of Slavonic Studies at the University of Nottingham as a point of comparison (access to the more recent results from Sheffield was no longer possible). The results give a tentative indication of differences in achievement, with the following caveats: final degree results include marks for non-language courses which are not streamed, as well as language courses; they also include results from second-year courses for which the former beginners' language courses are assessed differently from the post A-level language courses; finally, of course, the samples are very small and would be subject to the influence of countless variables (see Figures 3 and 4).

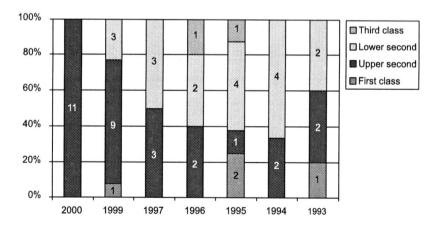

Figure 3: Percentage of post-A level students achieving first, upper or lower second and third class degrees at the Russian/Slavonic Studies departments of two British universities (values on chart refer to actual number of students)

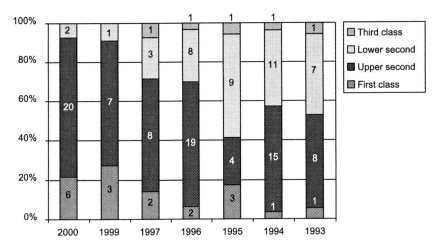

Figure 4: Percentage of *ab initio* students achieving first, upper or lower second and third class degrees at the Russian/Slavonic Studies departments of two British universities (values on chart refer to actual number of students)

The charts show that in five out of seven years, a higher percentage of former *ab initio* students than post-A level students obtain first class degrees, and in five out of seven years, a higher percentage of former *ab initio* students than post-A level students obtain upper second class degrees. This spread is offset by the fact that in three out of five years where third class degrees were awarded, a higher percentage of *ab initio* students than students with A Level achieve a third class degree.

Given that the degree results represent a single measure of outcome, the evidence they present needs to be corroborated by other sources. Satisfaction with a course may have a bearing on student performance. For this reason student course evaluation questionnaires (CEQs) for language modules from first to final year for the periods 1996/97 and 1995/96 were examined. The data obtained from the CEQs needs to be regarded only as a broad indicator of student opinion. The department produces a digest of the CEQs for each academic year, giving the average score per question and quoting some of the most useful comments, and this has been the source used. (See Appendix for an example of a blank CEQ.) The CEQ takes the same format for all language modules. The first question is: 'How do you rate the general quality of the course?'. For each module an overall average score was produced for comparison with the average rating of question one, and the lowest scoring question was noted. From these results only a very small difference in course satisfaction could be discerned between the *ab initio* modules and post-A level modules, streamed separately for the first two years, but most significantly, for both academic sessions studied, the first year *ab initio* course rated higher than the first year course for students with A level. For the second-year modules, this difference reversed itself, and final-year courses generally rated higher than first or second-year courses (See Figures 5 and 6).

The CEQ findings can be further explained by looking at the question which scored lowest on average for each module. It is significant that for both academic years, the lowest-scoring question for all first year courses and for the second-year post A level translation module was number nine: 'Was the pace of the course right for you?' On average it scored between two (not very good) and three (good). This could mean either too fast or too slow; additional comments added to the CEQs indicate that for the post-A Level courses the low score means too slow and for the *ab initio* courses, too fast.

Course description	Average general quality rating (score for question 1)	Overall average score (scores for all questions)
Year One: Post-A level *ab initio*	3 4.1	3.3 3.59
Year Two post-A level: Translation Comprehension	3.6 3	3.59 3.11
Year Two former *ab initio*: Translation Comprehension	3.5 3.3	3.43 3.09
Year Four (streams merged): Translation Comprehension	4.4 3.9	4.19 3.92

Figure 5: CEQ results for session 1996/97

Course description	Average general quality rating	Overall average score
Year One: Post-A level *ab initio*	3.4 4	3.36 3.69
Year Two post-A level: Translation Comprehension	4.3 4.0	4.01 4.5
Year Two former *ab initio:* Translation Comprehension	3.4 3.1	3.37 3.48
Year Four (streams merged): Translation i Translation ii Comprehension	3.7 4.3 4	3.6 4.14 3.47

Figure 6: CEQ results for session 1995/96

3.2   *The evidence from staff*

A questionnaire sent round to the staff involved in language teaching revealed some opinions which, if not actively reinforcing the evidence from the students, did not contradict it. (See Appendix for questionnaire.) Four lecturers were questioned, of whom three had at some time in the last six years been involved in post-A level and *ab initio* teaching at all levels. A wide range of answers presented itself. To the statement: 'In my experience first-year post-A level students are usually highly motivated in language classes', one lecturer responded with a rating of four; one remained neutral with a three, commenting that it depends on the individual and the group, and one strongly disagreed. First year *ab initio* students received a generally higher rating for motivation. A statement about progress made by second-year post-A level students elicited a rather lukewarm response, with two lecturers giving no more than the neutral three, and the third only two. In contrast, a statement referring to progress made by the second-year former beginners was rated four by both the lecturers with experience of this cohort. Finally, all four lecturers agreed or strongly agreed with the two last statements claiming that there was no difference in proficiency or motivation between final-year former A level and former *ab initio* students. Here there is an indication that, as was seen in the national picture, where problems exist they come within the first two years of the degree course. This concurs with the findings of the CEQs.

4 The outcome

The evidence presented above has often been conflicting, unrepresentative in some cases and very general in others, but a tentative conclusion may be drawn from it. It appears that students who start Russian from scratch at university progress faster and perform slightly better than students who enter with A level Russian. No real comment may be made about motivation in general. The evidence from the university case study indicates that post-A level entrants are less satisfied with their first years of university study, but there is nothing to propose what the national trend may be. Most significantly, even when the final degree results show little difference between cohorts, there is still an indication that this is in spite of potential earlier problems.

5 The reasons

Three hypotheses present themselves as explanations. Firstly, the university experience may be failing students who enter with A level Russian. Secondly, the school experience may be failing these students. Thirdly, a more politically acceptable option is that there may be a link between rate of progress and time spent learning a language. It should be stressed that none of these hypotheses are mutually exclusive.

5.1   The university experience

Evidence gathered largely from students and from TQA reports, whose focus is designed to be solely on university provision, supports the hypothesis that the university experience does not serve students with A level Russian as well as it does those who start *ab initio*. CEQs show a degree of dissatisfaction with early post-A level language courses; TQA reports highlight the first two years as a potential trouble spot for this sector of students while streaming is in place. When this evidence is examined next to final degree results, a link is suggested between disappointment and demotivation in the first two years and a less brilliant final achievement. Coleman's statistics (1996) presented in Figure 1 are an interesting counterpoint to the hypothesis, since they suggest that final-year post-A level students end up more proficient than final-year former beginners. The question then arises: why do Coleman's findings contradict trends in degree results? One possible explanation is that his C-Test is an indicator of a certain level of proficiency which may or may not correspond to final degree level in the universities tested; in other words, if this were the case, then **final degree level** would not be exactly the same in different universities.[2] Another possible explanation is that the institutionally neutral C-Test may not take account of other factors, such as motivation. Exactly how the university experience may be failing the post-A level entrants is beyond the bounds of this study; a number of factors may be responsible, such as difficulties of curriculum design, timetabling, staff resources and numbers of students, but without further research it is impossible to say.

5.2   *The school experience*

Another perspective on the issues raised in this study is that if post-A level students underperform at university, it is because of deficiencies in the school provision of Russian. In this area only anecdotal evidence was uncovered. Nevertheless, this anecdotal evidence, from interviews with university lecturers, points to matters for concern which need to be investigated by further research. There apparently exists a view, not uncommon amongst university teachers of Russian, that the A level Russian syllabus is inadequate for meeting entry requirements to a post-A level degree programme. Mention was made of bad linguistic habits formed during study for A level which the syllabus does not prevent, and these are then hard to correct at university, thus handicapping the students. It was suggested that the students themselves sometimes make hasty assumptions about their knowledge of the language; there have been cases of students protesting at studying material at university which they have ostensibly covered at school, while practice shows that the material has been imperfectly learned. Such a situation creates a gulf between the learners and the teachers. The inverse has also been known to occur, when staff assume that A level indicates a higher level of proficiency than has been attained in practice.

It was also asserted that because relatively few schools offer Russian to A level, the universities have a very small sample of post-A level applicants to consider for acceptance. Comparison was drawn between an entrant with a grade C at A level Russian, no other languages and a shaky grasp of the subject, and an entrant with A grades in one or more languages at A level, but who is adventurous and motivated enough to want to start another language from scratch and who may well be a better linguist. In a hypothetical case such as this, it would not be surprising should the *ab initio* learner perform better by final degree level. There is a potentially serious issue to be addressed behind these personal comments. Should there in fact be a mismatch between secondary and tertiary provision of Russian, there arises the question of whether to change the pace of the former or the latter to enable a smoother transition. The new developments for A and AS levels will also impact on this matter.

5.3   The 'slow down' hypothesis

A third, less politically sensitive, hypothesis is proposed, which does not challenge existing pedagogical practice. It draws on the findings of Coleman's survey (1996), from which, in my interpretation, the results presented above in Figure 2 and his additional corroborating evidence suggest that progress in language learning may not be proportional to the time spent learning; in other words, it becomes harder to make progress at more advanced levels. This would account for the apparent frustration of some first and second-year post-A level students that their courses seem to move at a sedate pace. The hypothesis that progress slows after a certain number of years of learning and does not pick up again until a few years later may be supported by research into links between age and language learning. Asher and Price (1967) found that, contrary to the popular belief that the younger one starts to learn a foreign language the quicker one will become proficient, adults are superior to children of any age group. On this basis, students who start Russian *ab initio* at university, and who are therefore at least eighteen years old, have age as an advantage over those students who began learning the language at school between the ages of eleven and sixteen. Neither would *ab initio* students be subject to the rallentando undergone by the post-A level students, as they would still be at the steep point of their learning curve for their university career; it seems that sheer momentum might carry them to greater achievement at final degree level. The 'slow down' hypothesis is interesting in that slow progress and underperformance of post-A level entrants would then have to be accepted as a natural occurrence which university teaching could not significantly influence.

6   Implications of the study

Whatever the reasons for the trend that *ab initio* students progress faster and perform slightly better than post-A level students, one salient issue emerges from the present study. Both final degree results and progress and satisfaction throughout the degree course have been considered here. Evidence from the TQA reports and from the university case study shows that even where the end result may not indicate any significant advantage of one cohort over the other, dissatisfaction and poor progress may occur in the early years of university study. The question is therefore one of focus: is it acceptable to focus on final achievement only and use that as an indicator of the success of a teaching programme? Most universities, I am sure, would disagree; some, however, may find it hard to put their beliefs into practice. If either the school experience hypothesis or the 'slow down' hypothesis can be proven, many universities may find that they have a much harder job to do with post-A level entrants, resulting in less impressive progress or student satisfaction. Nevertheless, it is clearly the responsibility of universities to keep all their students challenged and motivated and to stimulate progress at all levels.

7 Concluding remarks

The limitations of the evidence presented must be stressed: the overall picture has been based on very small sample sizes, which may not be representative of the whole sector. It has also been based on generalised statements, cross-sectional studies, averages and summaries; in particular, many of the comments in the TQA reports refer only to one year; degree results constitute marks from non-language courses as well as language courses. No account has been taken of variables such as the difference in provision at different institutions, factors influencing the quality of student entrants in various years, changes in the financial situation of higher education generally and departments of Russian specifically. Certain political considerations may have affected evidence from teaching staff and many affective considerations may have influenced student responses to CEQs. What is more, no mention has been made of students who enter university with GCSE Russian and whether they are able to choose which stream to enter.

Nevertheless, despite much conflicting evidence, the study has discovered the existence of a trend that *ab initio* students do slightly better than their more experienced fellow students and that problems involved in the early streaming of the two cohorts is more likely to have an adverse effect on the post-A level students. Further research is needed to separate and confirm or deny the many related issues raised by this study, the findings of which would without doubt be of enormous significance for the teaching of Russian at university.

Notes

1 Muckle, 1994, found 34 in the session 1991/92; since then at least one Department of Russian has been closed down due to financial cutbacks (University of Bangor). HEFCE assessed 28 institutions in England and Northern Ireland for Teaching Quality in Russian and Slavonic Studies in 1995/96. There are probably about half a dozen more institutions offering Russian in Wales and Scotland.

2 Coleman's view of this possibility (1996) is that without desiring recourse to league tables, there should be a nationally accepted way of measuring linguistic proficiency and an acknowledgement of which level on that scale each degree programme aims to achieve.

References

Asher, J. and Price, B. (1967) 'The learning strategy of total physical response: some age differences' in *Child development*, 38: 1219–1227.

Coleman, J. (1996) *Studying languages: a survey of British and European students.* London: CILT.

Gardner, R. and Lambert, W. (1972) *Attitudes and motivation in second language learning.* Rowley, Mass: Newbury House Publishers.

Grotjahn, R. (1996) *Der C-Test. Theoretische Grundlagen und praktische Anwendungen.* Vol. 3. Bochum: Brockmeyer.

HEFCE, (1996) *Quality assessment of Russian and Eastern European languages and studies 1995–6: subject overview report.* QO 7/96. HEFCE.

HEFCE, (1995–6) *Quality assessment reports for individual universities in Russian and Eastern European languages and studies and modern languages.* www.niss.ac.uk/hefce/qar/

Jones, J., Harris, A. and Putt, G. (1990) 'Streaming in first-year university classes' in *Studies in Higher Education* 15 (1): 21–30.

Muckle, J. (1995) 'Starting Russian at university: expectations and reactions of students' in *Rusistika*, 11: 43–49.

Muckle, J. (1994) 'Survey of schools, polytechnics and universities where Russian is taught' in *Educational Research*, 36 (1): 39–50.

Thompson, I. (1996) 'Assessing foreign language skills: data from Russian' in *Modern Language Journal*, 80: 47–65.

University of Sheffield (1995) *Department of Russian and Slavonic Studies: Teaching Quality Assessment Self-Assessment statement.*

Appendix

Questionnaire sent to teaching staff in the University of Sheffield Department of Russian and Slavonic Studies.

1. Which language courses do you currently teach? Please state course title and level.
2. Which language courses have you taught in the past? Please state course title and level.

Please indicate agreement/disagreement with the following statements (5 = strongly agree, 1 = strongly disagree) and add comments if appropriate:

3. In my experience, first-year post-A level students are usually highly motivated in language classes.
4. In my experience, first-year *ab initio* students are usually highly motivated in language classes.
5. In my experience, second-year A level students make significant progress in language on their first year.
6. In my experience, second-year ex-beginners make significant progress in language on their first year.
7. In my experience, there is no difference in language proficiency between final-year A level students and final-year ex-beginners.
8. In my experience, there is no difference in motivation between final-year A level students and final-year ex-beginners.

University of Sheffield Department of Russian and Slavonic Studies: Student Course Evaluation Questionnaire.

HOW TO USE THE QUESTIONNAIRE

> 5 = Excellent
> 4 = Very Good
> 3 = Good
> 2 = Not Very Good
> 1 = Bad

This questionnaire is **anonymous.**

1. How do you rate the general quality of the course?
2. Were the classes clearly conducted?
3. How relevant did you find the classes to the stated aims of the course?
4. If handouts were provided, how useful were they?
5. Was the teacher easy to hear and understand?

6. Was the use of chalkboard, OHP, or other audio-visual aids satisfactory and appropriate to the nature of the course?
7. Was the level of student participation appropriate to the nature of the course?
8. How useful did you find written or oral feedback on work done?
9. Was the pace of the course right for you? (Comment overleaf, if necessary, indicating whether too fast/slow)
10. Given the format and time constraints of the course, how adequate was the coverage of the subject concerned?

Dropping out, opting out or staying in: reasons for continuation and non-continuation of German on an Institution-Wide Languages Programme

Nicola Reimann ● *University of Sunderland*

1 Introduction

A large number of institutions of higher education (HE) operate Institution-Wide Languages Programmes (IWLPs) which allow students of virtually all disciplines to take up or continue learning a foreign language alongside the study of their main subjects. Modularisation and credit accumulation and transfer have further encouraged the existence of such programmes. German is one of the most widely available languages on IWLPs, particularly at beginner and post-GCSE level (Pilkington, 1997). Many of these programmes, however, fall short of the aims which they set out to achieve since a large proportion of students who register on IWLPs discontinue foreign language study, either by not completing individual language modules or by not pursuing the study of a language beyond a limited period and/or until a considerable level of competence has been achieved.

The research which is summarised in this article has investigated non-continuation on the IWLP of one university. The example of German has been used as a way of capturing the process of studying a language on an IWLP. The goal of the study was to describe and understand whether there are any specific differences between students who discontinue the study of German and those who persist. Particular attention was given to the role of students' perceptions of the classroom and of language-learning motivation for continuation and non-continuation and whether any particular events, experiences, feelings or strategies contribute to the decision to drop out or to persist.

2 Insights from the literature

Three distinct areas of literature have informed the research: studies specifically investigating drop-out from L2 learning (from now on called language drop-out), literature on L2 motivation as well as studies dealing with drop-out from non-compulsory education, particularly from higher education in the UK (McGivney, 1996, Mortgaat, 1996, Ozga and Sukhnandan, 1997, Yorke *et al*, 1997). The latter provided insights of a general nature, e.g. regarding issues of definition and approach, whereas the fomer areas were of more direct relevance.

Attitudes and motivation stand out as significant for an understanding of the drop-out phenomenon. A relatively recent upsurge in interest in L2 motivation (Crookes and Schmidt, 1991, Oxford and Shearin, 1994, Dörnyei, 1994) has resulted in new approaches and models of L2 motivation which have contributed to the conceptualisation of non-continuation and its location within a temporal sequence. Tremblay and Gardner (1995), for instance, classify persistence as one component of motivated behaviour which is influenced by motivational antecedents. In two other recent models of L2 motivation, non-continuation is conceptualised as one possible outcome of the entire motivational process (Williams and Burden, 1997, Dörnyei and Ottó, 1998).

Previous language drop-out studies have identified a multitude of reasons and factors impacting on drop-out. Some studies, for instance, have found drop-outs to display lower levels of motivation, to be less integratively and/or more instrumentally motivated[1] (Gardner and Smythe, 1975, Clément, Smythe and Gardner, 1978, Myers, 1996). The kind of reasons identified depend to a large extent on the theoretical background of each study. Research carried out on the basis of motivation theory, for instance, has tended to confirm differences in motivational type as decisive for language drop-out (*ibid*), whereas action research carried out by teachers has emphasised the impact of classroom factors such as difficulty, mixed nature of classes and dissatisfaction with syllabus and methodology (Rowsell, 1990, Aplin, 1991 a and b, Ball, 1993, 1994). In addition, personal factors, i.e. differences in ability and aptitude (Bartley, 1969, 1970, Sidwell, 1980), grades and age when starting foreign language study (Ramage, 1990) have all been found to be responsible for drop-out, as have more external factors, such as academic workload (Frahm and Rippel, 1988, Myers, 1996), taking a language as a college requirement (Ramage, 1990), extra-curricular activities (Frahm and Rippel, 1988), home, work and financial difficulties (Ball, 1993, 1994). Although extremely different contexts have been investigated, such as higher, adult and further education in a number of countries, institutions and classrooms, very few of the studies explicitly deal with the context and its influence on the findings. They also do not contain any classroom observations nor make any other attempts to investigate the impact of the classroom in any in-depth manner. Survey questionnaires and test batteries have been the preferred instruments and, with the notable exception of Rowsell (1990), all studies interpret student responses as factual, objective information. Few studies acknowledge the longitudinal nature of drop-out (Bartley, 1970, Gardner and Smythe, 1975, Rowsell, 1990), but this tends to be done merely by collecting data twice. Insight into drop-out as a process and into the nature of decision making can hardly be gained from the literature.

3 Methodology

The present study makes a specific contribution to the understanding of language drop-out by taking a case study approach which draws on the ethnographic[2] tradition and includes longitudinal data collection and classroom observation. Other studies of non-continuation (Rowsell, 1990, Ozgan and Sukhnandan, 1997) have demonstrated that qualitative methods and the consideration of context and perceptions can lead to findings which are very different from those of survey methodology.

In the present study, non-continuation is investigated as a phenomenon which is set within a specific institutional and classroom culture and certain aspects of this culture are selected for investigation and analysis. The study comprises ethnographic elements in its attention to the context in which non-continuation occurs, in its attempts to adopt as closely as possible the perspective of the students concerned and in the way in which explanation and understanding are grounded in the data themselves rather than being derived from a predetermined hypothesis. It is a case study because of its narrower focus, the multiplicity of evidence and data-gathering techniques used, including quantitative data for triangulation[3] purposes, and the way in which the understanding which is gained is intended to illuminate issues which are also relevant for other IWLPs. Case studies tend to be longitudinal in design since an in-depth understanding can only be gained by gradual immersion and detailed data collection from a multitude of sources and does not lend itself to once-off, speedy data collection. The present study's longitudinality is also due to a conceptualisation of (non-)continuation which emphasises it being the result of a process rather than a static phenomenon.

4 Overview of the study

The study was carried out between September 1996 and July 1997. At the university under investigation, IWLP modules in several languages were available to students across the entire university as well as to members of staff and the general public. The provision was fully modularised and semesterised and German could be taken from *ab initio* to post-A level and throughout the entire duration of students' degree courses. The integration of language modules into programmes of study was subject to discipline-specific programme regulations, although in theory most programmes were supposed to reserve twenty compulsory credits per year for an elective module which could be chosen from a variety of subjects, including languages. Alternatively, students were able to take a language as an additional module on top of their compulsory credit requirements. All German IWLP modules consisted of three hours contact time and, with the exception of beginners' modules, took place over two semesters. Assessment covered all four skills and was either exclusively continuous or a combination of continuous assessment with end-of-year examinations.

In order to investigate non-continuation, non-continuing students needed to be identified; however, the impossibility of compiling objective registration and (non-)continuation figures soon became obvious. For the purposes of the research, attempts were made to obtain the most comprehensive record possible. Since ascertaining the influence of the classroom was an important aim of the study, particular care was taken to include every student who attended, even if it was only for an extremely brief period.

As a result of close contact with the data, three main categories of students were established. **Stay-ins** are those students who completed a module during the academic year under investigation. Students in the **drop-out** category attended a module a least once and withdrew or stopped attending while it was still in progress. Students who registered, but dropped out without ever attending any classes, are listed separately. So are students who withdrew for reasons unrelated to the language module, such as maternity leave, exchange students returning to their home universities or students dropping out of HE altogether. The latter type of non-continuing students is labelled 'others'. **Opt-outs**, i.e. the third major category, are students who completed a German module in the academic year prior to the investigation, but did not progress to the subsequent module.

The following four German modules (see Figure 1) were investigated since they had tended to attract the highest drop-out rates in the past.

Linguistic level	Prerequisites	Duration in semesters	Credits
Beginners, part 1	No previous knowledge of German	1	10
Lower-intermediate	GCSE, grade C or lower or Beginners, part 2	2	20
Upper-intermediate	GCSE, grade A or B or Lower-intermediate (also requirement for students admitted to German degree without A level)	2	20
Advanced 1	A level or Upper-intermediate	2	20

Figure 1: German modules under investigation

Initially, every student who registered for German received a pre-course questionnaire asking for background information, motives for studying German, expectations, intentions, hopes and fears (see Figure 2). Statistical information on non-continuation was compiled for each of the four modules. Individual groups of students taking the four modules and their classrooms were observed regularly for two or three hours, weekly in the first semester, fortnightly in semester two in the case of the lower and upper-intermediate modules. While observing classes, fieldnotes were taken and students provided regular feedback on the learning experience by writing short entries for their learner diaries and completing after-class questionnaires[+] in alternate weeks. When students dropped out, they were sent a questionnaire focusing on reasons for drop-out and were asked to be interviewed as well. Opt-outs were sent a questionnaire similar to the one drop-outs received and were also interviewed if they consented; stay-ins were only interviewed. Interviews were also conducted with the three main module teachers. All interviews were unstructured and in-depth.

136   LANGUAGE-LEARNING FUTURES

All students taking German during academic year under investigation	Module statistics Pre-course questionnaires
One group of students for each module	Observations Diaries After-class questionnaires
Drop-outs	Drop-out questionnaires Drop-out interviews
Opt-outs	Opt-out questionnaires Opt-out interviews
Stay-ins	Stay-in interviews
Teachers	Teacher interviews

Figure 2: Data

5 Findings

5.1 Non-continuation statistics

Registration and (non-)continuation figures form the baseline data for the investigation (see Figure 3)and illustrate the actual extent of non-continuation. It has to be borne in mind that this is a case study and no attempts are made to generalise and regard these figures as representative in any way.

	Beg.	Lower intermed.	Upper intermed.	Advanced	Overall
Students overall	67	73	36	9	185
Attending students	53	65	33	7	158
Registered, non-attending students	14	8	3	2	27

Figure 3: Number of students on modules

As can be seen from the raw figures, student uptake on the two lower-level modules was much higher than on the upper-intermediate module, and it was extremely low on the advanced module. Particularly on the lower levels, a considerable number of students registered for a German module without ever attending.

	Beg.	Lower intermed.	Upper intermed.	Advanced	Overall
Based on attending students*	51%	59%	31%	50%	50%
Based on registered and attending students*	64%	63%	37%	67%	58%

* excluding others (students who left the university, e.g. exchange students, university drop-outs, maternity leave etc)

Figure 4: Drop-out rate

In Figure 4, the percentages illustrate first and foremost the alarming extent of non-continuation. Despite considerable variation in original registration and attendance figures, drop-out rates were similar for three of the four modules, with the exception of upper-intermediate German. Over half of all students on these modules eventually dropped out, with some variation depending on who is counted as an original module participant. The drop-out rate in the observed groups was slightly lower, but this might be a direct consequence of being observed.

Student attendance, and therefore the exact point at which drop-outs discontinued their respective German module, was also recorded during classroom observations. A considerable amount of drop-out took place within the initial weeks and sessions of a module. Drop-out culminated within weeks 1–3 or after attending one or two sessions, then eased off in week 4–6 or after attending three to four sessions and finally turned into a small trickle for the remainder of the sessions. After week 6 the majority of drop-outs had left and far fewer students decided half-way through the module that they would not continue the study of German. The data suggest that the early experiences on the module, or elsewhere, must be particularly significant in their influence on non-continuation.

Opt-out figures show a similar trend to those on drop-out, i.e. a large proportion of students who completed a German module during the previous academic year did not continue the study of the language. Figures 5 and 6 also list those students who initially attended the subsequent module, but decided later on to drop it.

	Ex-beg.	Ex-low. intermed.	Ex-up. intermed.	Ex-adv.	Overall
Completers previous year	28	23	7	4	62
Continuing students	9	5	0	2	16
Opt-outs	11	15	4	1	31
Continuing students who dropped out later on (drop-outs)	6	1	1	1	9
Others	2	2	2	0	6

Figure 5: Opt-outs

	Ex-beg.	Ex-low. intermed.	Ex-up. intermed.	Ex-adv.	Overall
Based on opt-outs*	42%	71%	80%	25%	55%
Based on opt-outs and drop-outs*	65%	76%	100%	50%	71%

* excluding 'others' (students who left the university, e.g. exchange students, university drop-outs, maternity leave etc)

Figure 6: Opt-out rate

Over half of the students who had already completed a German module on the IWLP did not continue the study of German. Coupled with the high average drop-out rate, the equally high numbers of opt-outs imply that very few students who initially choose to take German persist in the study of the language for any substantial amount of time. As approximately half of the students discontinue a module while it is in progress (drop-out) and of those who complete a module, over half do not go on to the next one (opt-out), those students who pursue the language throughout their entire degree or most of it represent an extremely small minority.

5.2 Reasons for non-continuation

Data analysis concentrated on the identification of themes within the diaries and interviews. These were compared to responses to questionnaire items and interpreted on the background of classroom observations. This procedure resulted in the following reasons for non-continuation:

- priority of main subject;
- workload of main subject;
- credit considerations;
- difficulty of learning German;
- workload of German;
- timetable problems;
- coping with being a university student;
- misinformation and unfortunate circumstances;
- satisfaction with acquired language skills;
- absence from classes.

Not all of the reasons listed above are of equal importance and the following discussion focuses on those reasons which were confirmed by both interview and questionnaire data.

5.3   Priority of main subject

The priority of the main degree subject is the most significant influence on non-continuation. Priority and workload are, of course, closely inter-related as the amount of work and effort expended for a subject depends to a large extent on the priority it is given. The most striking finding is that drop-outs view their higher education predominantly as having to fulfil module requirements, gain good marks and the best possible degree classification, whereas actual learning is less relevant for them. Despite drop-outs' interest in German, it is not a priority due to the absence of extrinsic rewards connected to the language. This absence of extrinsic rewards is related to the status of the language module both within students' programmes and within the modular credit scheme as a whole. When talking about German, drop-outs depict language learning as a leisure pursuit, a hobby and personal interest which is contrasted with the academic and vocational benefits of the main programme. German and the degree are perceived to be unrelated to each other and are deliberately kept separate. Although some drop-outs also stress their intrinsic interest in their main subject, it is predominantly extrinsic aspects which make them prioritise in favour of their degree subject and at the expense of German. Drop-out is a result of the dilemma between what is regarded as the purely personal benefit of learning German and the perception that the time and effort spent on German prevents the achievement of extrinsic rewards for the degree.

5.4   *Workload*

While drop-outs tend to stress the priority of their main subject, opt-outs dwell on the workload which is involved when combining the study of German with that of their main subject. This is not surprising since opt-outs have had some experience of the workload by completing at least one German module in the previous academic year. Information on what students really do for their modules is not available, but it can be assumed that individual students carry out very different amounts of work. However, it is the perception and anticipation of workload rather than the actual experience of a specific workload which has an impact on students' decision not to continue with the language. Myers's (1996) study, which also identifies workload as the most important reason for drop-out from an IWLP, does not draw attention to the perceptual nature of workload.

When talking about workload, it is the workload of their main subject more than that of German which is repeatedly mentioned by drop-outs, but pre-course questionnaires also illustrate students' unrealistically low expectations regarding the workload of their German modules (see Figure 7).

	0–15 min	15–30 min	30–60 min	60–120 min	120–180 min	180–240 min	over 240 min
Stay-ins			7.5%	46.3%	29.9%	10.4%	6%
Drop-outs	1.6%	7.9%	7.9%	47.6%	20.6%	11.1%	3.2%
All students	0.8%	3.8%	7.7%	46.9%	25.4%	10.8%	4.6%

Figure 7: Anticipated weekly study time for German

While module regulations stipulate approximately three hours of self study per week, the majority of students expect between one and two hours. Drop-outs estimate a somewhat lower study time for German than stay-ins; it must be noted, however, that these differences are not statistically significant.

Whereas stay-ins consider the workload of German to be manageable, non-continuing students find themselves unable to reconcile the workload of their main subject with that of German. In their diaries, all students display considerable awareness of the necessity of regular and sufficient work for language learning and of the way in which the continuity of effort distinguishes languages from other subjects. While the work for students' main subjects is described as following a wave-like pattern, the continuous nature of the work required for German makes it appear never-ending, and this apparent incompatibility between German and the degree subject contributes to non-continuation. For some stay-ins, on the other hand, it is precisely the regular and continuous nature of the work for German which makes it easier rather than more difficult to fit it around their main subjects.

It is not only the different nature and pattern of the work which appears to make the degree subject incompatible with German. Non-continuing students regard German modules as difficult (see 5.5 below) and therefore more work-intensive than other modules. The interview data also suggest that the majority of opt-outs may not employ appropriate (language-)learning strategies and therefore invest a disproportionate amount of time into the study of German without achieving satisfactory results. Stay-ins, on the other hand, feel that the amount of learning which takes place makes their effort worthwhile. They are realistic in their expectations of what can be achieved and therefore accept doing less in times of stress instead of giving up German altogether. A particularly successful strategy is deliberately taking the language as an accredited module with a view to reducing overall workload and taking German as seriously as possible.

5.5   *Difficulty of learning German*

The perceived difficulty of the German module is the only classroom-related reason for non-continuation consistently brought up by various types of data. Other language drop-out studies have also identified difficulty as a significant factor for drop-out (Rowsell, 1990, Myers, 1996). Diary data illustrate that difficulty is on students' minds from beginning to end of the module. According to the interviews, a number of influences contribute to perceptions of difficulty and therefore to non-continuation. Drop-outs express an acute desire for understanding the rules of the language and experience frustration when this cannot be achieved. The vague and unspecified concept of 'the basics', which features in several interviews, embodies drop-outs' conviction that a certain body of knowledge exists which needs to be grasped before being able to move on and eventually master the language. As students fail to understand the rules of the language and their teacher's explanations, this is a cause for drop-out.

Another aspect of perceived difficulty is the complexity of reading and listening texts as well as teacher target-language use in the classroom. Drop-outs expect complete, native-like comprehension and instead of regarding comprehension problems as a normal element of language use and a pathway to language learning, non-comprehension of any kind is appropriated with having been allocated to the wrong level module. Drop-outs are unwilling to accept confusion, uncertainty and imperfection, errors and inaccuracies as integral components of learning. They do not like taking risks and appear to be unfamiliar with appropriate comprehension and language-learning strategies. Although some stay-ins experience difficulties much in the same way as non-continuing students, they are more likely to regard difficulty as a positive challenge and do not expect perfect mastery, control and native-like comprehension as some of the drop-outs do.

Due to the unstructured nature of the observation data, text and task difficulty were not measured and related to student perceptions, but there is some indication that the perceived difficulty may be, at least to some extent, due to teacher behaviour and certain methodological procedures. For instance, whenever students were required to move immediately from comprehension to production, this was experienced as pressure to perform and interpreted as too difficult. Similarly, when authentic or semi-authentic texts were approached in a word-by-word fashion without focusing on gist comprehension first, students expressed frustration and described these classes as extremely difficult. However, students' judgements of the overall level of difficulty did not necessarily coincide with the observations and perceptions of the researcher. They frequently complained of having been allocated to the wrong level module, while they appeared to be coping well. Students were also more likely to attribute their problems to the difficulty of the language and language learning overall, whereas the researcher tended to make certain actions and methodological decisions by the teacher responsible. However, many other influences in addition to teacher behaviour and methodology seem to contribute to the overall impression of the level of difficulty of a specific module. Students base their decision to continue or discontinue the study of German on judgements of difficulty which do not appear to be exclusively related to some measurable objective difficulty. The exact causes of individual perceptions of difficulty deserve further investigation.

5.6   The role of the classroom experience

Apart from difficulty, no other classroom-related reasons for non-continuation emerged. When students were asked in after-class questionnaires to rate the quality of their classes, there were no differences of statistical significance between drop-outs and stay-ins. In the drop-out and opt-out questionnaires, most respondents stated that the experience on their German module and its quality had not been an influence on their decision to discontinue the study of the language (see Figures 8 and 9).

In what way has your experience on the German module and its quality been an influence on your decision not to continue with German?

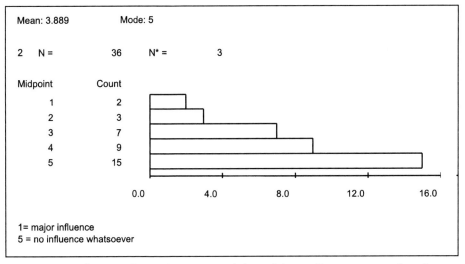

Figure 8: Influence of experience on module and its quality on non-continuation according to drop-out questionnaires

In what way has your experience on the German module and its quality been an influence on your decision not to continue with German?

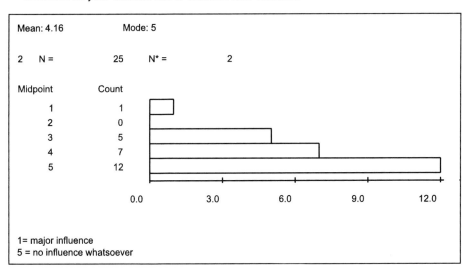

Figure 9: Influence of experience on module and its quality on non-continuation according to opt-out questionnaires

Only a very small minority of drop-outs explicitly make the classroom experience responsible for non-continuation. These tend to be those students who perceive the module as too difficult. The majority of stay-ins, drop-outs and opt-outs, however, stress their enjoyment of the classes. Enjoyment is a recurrent interview theme, although there is considerable variation between individual students as to what is liked and disliked. The enjoyment of stay-ins as expressed in the interviews appears to be somewhat more pronounced than that of non-continuing students, but it is impossible to quantify the evidence due to its qualitative nature. Even if there is a difference, drop-outs and opt-outs stress and agree that enjoyment alone does not guarantee continuation.

Although the classroom experience does not have a direct impact on non-continuation, certain critical areas are salient in most students' experiences and perceptions of the language classroom. The majority of students have very strong opinions, both positive and negative, about teacher target-language use, accuracy and grammar, speaking and participation as well as the use of complex texts. Students are particularly sensitive to the way in which these areas are handled in the classroom and experiences related to these areas may trigger the decision to discontinue the study of German, particularly if they contribute to the perception of difficulty. The small number of drop-outs who discontinued German for classroom-related reasons stated that too much teacher target-language use, an excessive emphasis on accuracy, confusing grammar teaching, too little speaking and participation as well as the use of long and complex texts contributed to their decision.

5.7   The role of motivation

According to pre-course questionnaires stay-ins are more integratively motivated than non-continuing students. The pre-course questionnaires also provide some evidence that both drop-outs and stay-ins have more extrinsic than intrinsic motives for taking German; at the same time, these two groups of students stress their strong intrinsic motives for German in the interviews.

The importance of extrinsic rewards for all students, in particular their orientation towards the best possible degree classification, has already been mentioned above. Although drop-outs want to learn German for its own sake, it is their motivation for their degree programme and their concept of the role of linguistic skills for their higher education which have much more impact on continuation than their specific motivation for German. Whereas non-continuing students regard German and their main subject as entirely separate, for stay-ins German is a much more integral part of their higher education. This is why stay-ins are more likely to take German as an accredited module whose marks and credits count towards their degree. The combination of intrinsic and extrinsic motives for learning German is therefore most conducive for continuation. This points to the theory of self-determination and the way in which it is suited to explaining language drop-out as a feature of motivation within an institutional setting. According to Deci and Ryan (1985), extrinsic rewards which are chosen under conditions allowing autonomy can be combined with or lead to intrinsic motivation (Dörnyei, 1998: 21).

5.8   *The role of the institutional context and modularity*

Non-continuation, including the relevance of motivation, can only be understood if the influence of the context is considered as well. The study has demonstrated that the institutional culture provides the framework and overarching context for student behaviour and perceptions and is much more important than the classroom context. The status of the language module is determined by its role within students' programmes of study and by students' interpretations and experiences of the modular system. Some students take German purely to make up credits, others take it in order to complement perceived shortcomings of a specific programme or, in the true spirit of the modular system (HEQC 1994), to add to their portfolio of skills. In students' minds, however, a number of reasons exist against German, such as the conviction that modules which are more closely related to the main subject will reinforce success on the degree, the necessity to fulfil pre- and co-requisites for other modules or to adhere to stipulations made by professional organisations in order to achieve accredited status, e.g. for future engineers or psychologists. According to interviews, fellow students and main subject lecturers tend to advise to concentrate on the degree. These considerations influence whether German is taken as an elective, an extra module or as a 'reserve' which can be used in case another module is failed.

The modular system is perceived by students as emphasising the achievement of extrinsic rewards. It fuels extrinsic motivation and encourages strategic decisions. In the modular market place, German competes with other subjects and credit considerations are much more decisive for continuation than interest in German and enjoyment of the classroom experience. This is why neither intrinsic nor integrative motivation alone are sufficient to prevent non-continuation of German.

6 Conclusion and implications

The present study has shown that non-continuation can only be adequately understood within the context in which it occurs. Rather than taking non-continuation as, for instance, a sign of teacher incompetence or an IWLP's failure to provide quality learning experiences, it is, at least partially, a reflection of the system of modularity and students' interpretation of credit accumulation and transfer. Extrinsic rewards and the goal of the best possible degree classification are the main motivators within the HE context, so that a positive reaction towards the classroom alone does not guarantee continuation. Only those students who drop out due to perceived difficulty make the classroom responsible for their decision. On the other hand, students who regard learning German as an integral component of their education as well as taking the language as an accredited module are least likely to drop out.

The study highlights the role of goal hierarchies and conflicts (Dörnyei and Ottó, 1998) and of the institutional context for the sustainment of motivation and the importance to include such factors into current models of L2 motivation. It also demonstrates a way in which self-determination theory (Deci and Ryan, 1985) can be applied to explain learning within an institutional setting. The need for further research which explores the relationship between perceptions of difficulty and classroom experience has also become obvious.

The study has a number of possible implications, ranging from classroom practice to institutional and national policy level. Since difficulty has been shown to be the only classroom factor which has a bearing on non-continuation, adequate placement of students is important, as are attempts to dissolve perceptions of extreme difficulty, e.g. by sensitive handling of teacher target-language use, accuracy and grammar, speaking and participation and the use of long and complex comprehension texts. Ultimately, however, maximum continuation will only be achieved if students can be made to regard language learning as a relevant and integral component of their education and become aware of the relevance of language skills for their main subject. It is hypothesised that this is best achieved by internationalising the HE curriculum and by closer co-operation between languages and other disciplines, resulting, for instance, in increased integration of language and culture-specific elements and content into non-language modules and programmes. Other desirable measures comprise a change in funding mechanisms with a view to making individual programmes less protective about their own students, a centrally organised timetable with dedicated slots for languages, institutional commitment to adequate pastoral care as well as systematic and continuous development of students' study and time-management skills. Above all, fostering an institutional culture which emphasises and promotes intrinsic motivation and self-determination will be crucial in reducing non-continuation on IWLPs.

Notes

1 According to the social psychological theory of motivation associated with Gardner and colleagues (e.g. Gardner, 1985, Gardner and MacIntyre, 1993), 'integrative' refers to the desire to learn an L2 in order to interact with speakers of the language and eventually become an integrated, valued member of the L2 community, whereas 'instrumental' motivation is the desire to learn the language for more pragmatic benefits, such as obtaining a job or getting promoted.

2 Ethnography has been defined as '... the study of the culture/characteristics of a group in real-world rather than laboratory settings. The researcher makes no attempt to isolate or manipulate the phenomena under investigation, and insights and generalisation emerge from close contact with the data rather than from a theory of language learning and use.' (Nunan, 1992: 55)

3 Triangulation refers to the 'use of two or more methods of data collection in the study of some aspect of human behaviour. (...) ... (T)riangular techniques in the social sciences attempt to map out, or explain more fully, the richness and complexity of human behaviour by studying it from more than one standpoint and, in doing so, by making use of both quantitative and qualitative data.' (Cohen and Manion, 1989: 269). Triangulation also contributes to the reliability and validity of a qualitative study such as the present one.

4 As students dropped out over the weeks, after-class questionnaires were increasingly received from stay-ins only. Therefore, little data allowing statistical comparison between drop-outs and stay-ins were available and analysis was only performed on the questionnaires completed in weeks 1 and 3.

References

Aplin, R. (1991a) 'The ones who got away: the views of those who opt out of languages' in *Language learning journal*, 4: 2–4.

Aplin, R. (1991b) 'Why do pupils opt out of foreign language courses? – a pilot study' in *Educational studies*, 17(1): 3–13.

Ball, C. (1993) *Modern language students in adult education. Why the high drop-out rate? What can we do to stem the tide? A survey of 52 students enrolled on modern language courses in Mid-Cheshire College and its Adult Education Centres in September 1992 who had dropped out by February 1993.* RSA Dip TFLA.

Ball, C. (1994) 'Modern language students in AE. Why the high drop-out rate? What can we do to stem the tide?' in *Netword* 16.

Bartley, D. E. (1969) 'A pilot study of aptitude and attitude factors in language drop-out' in *Journal of educational research*, 20: 48–55.

Bartley, D. E. (1970) 'The importance of the attitude factor in language drop-out: a preliminary investigation of group and sex differences' in *Foreign language annals*, 3: 383–393.

Clément, R., Smythe, P. C. and Gardner, R. C. (1978) 'Persistence in second-language study: motivational considerations' in *Canadian modern language review*, 34: 688–694.

Cohen, L. and Manion, L. (1989) *Research methods in education*. London, New York: Routledge.

Crookes, G. and Schmidt, R. W. (1991) 'Motivation: reopening the research agenda' in *Language learning*, 41(4): 469–512.

Deci, E. L. and Ryan, R. M. (1985) '*Intrinsic motivation and self-determination in human behavior*. New York: Plenum.

Dörnyei, Z. (1994) 'Motivation and motivating in the foreign language classroom' in *Modern language journal*, 78(3): 273–284.

Dörnyei, Z. (1998) 'Motivation and foreign language learning' in *Language teaching*, 31: 117–135.

Dörnyei, Z. and Ottó, I. (1998) 'Motivation in action: a process model of L2 motivation' in *Working papers in applied linguistics*, 4: 43–69. London: Thames Valley University.

Frahm, G. F. and Rippel, Z. I. B. (1988) 'The drop-out phenomenon: a study of mixed group ESP drop-outs in the Federal University of Parana' in Celani, M. A. A. *et al* (eds) *The Brazilian ESP project. An evaluation*. 137–142. Sao Paulo: Educ.

Gardner, R. (1985) *Social psychology and second language learning*. London: Edward Arnold.

Gardner, R. and MacIntyre, P. D. (1993) 'A student's contribution to second-language learning. Part II: Affective variables' in *Language teaching*, 26, 1–11.

Gardner, R. and Smythe, P. C. (1975) 'Motivation and second-language acquisition' in *Canadian modern language review*, 31(3): 218–230.

Higher Education Quality Council (HEQC) CAT Project (1994) *Choosing to change. Extending access, choice and mobility in higher education*. Published report, London: HEQC.

McGivney (1996) *Staying or leaving the course. Non-completion and retention of mature students in further and higher education*. Leicester: National Institute of Adult Continuing Education.

Mortgaat, J. L. (1996) *A study of drop-out in European higher education. Case studies of five countries*. Research report for the Council of Europe.

Myers, G. (1996) *Student drop-out and retention on the university language scheme. Project report in partial fulfilment of the requirements for the degreee of MA in further and higher education*. Unpublished report, Sheffield Hallam University, School of Education.

Nunan, D. (1992) *Research methods in language learning*. Cambridge: Cambridge University Press.

Oxford, R. and Shearin J. (1994) 'Language learning motivation: expanding the theoretical framework' in *Modern language journal*, 78(1): 12–28.

Ozga, R. and Sukhnandan, L. (1997) *Undergraduate non-completion. A report for the Higher Education Funding Council for England.* Bristol: Higher Education Funding Council for England (HEFCE).

Pilkington, R. (1997) *Survey of non-specialist language provision in further and higher education institutions in the United Kingdom research report as part of the TransLang project.* Preston: University of Central Lancashire.

Ramage, K. (1990) 'Motivational factors and persistence in foreign language study' in *Language Learning* 40(2): 189–219.

Rowsell, L. (1990) *Classroom factors pertaining to drop-out among adult ESL students: a constructivist analysis.* Unpublished PhD thesis, University of Lancaster.

Sidwell, D. (1980) 'A survey of modern language classes' in *Adult education*, 52: 309–331.

Tremblay, P. F. and Gardner, R. C. (1995) 'Expanding the motivation construct in language learning' in *Modern Language Learning*, 79(4): 505–518.

Williams, M. and Burden, R. L. (1997) *Psychology for language teachers: a social constructivist approach.* Cambridge. Cambridge University Press.

Yorke, M. (1997) *et al Undergraduate non-completion in England.* Final report of a research project commissioned by HEFCE (Bristol: Higher Education Funding Council of England (HEFCE).

Strategies for the development of multicultural competence in language learning

Inma Álvarez and Cecilia Garrido ● The Open University

1 Introduction

Over the past few years, the Open University (OU) has been involved in the development of a Spanish programme geared to students who want to learn the language at a distance. The task has been a challenge not only because of the obvious difficulties that learning a language at a distance poses, but also because Spanish is a language spoken in three continents, by 21 countries and by at least as many cultures. The teaching of culture is therefore at the core of the development of the OU Spanish courses. It is an integral part of the syllabus, the writing of the materials and the development of strategies that will enable students to interact effectively in a multicultural setting. This paper will explore the main issues relating to the development of a language programme that gives equal importance to linguistic and cultural content, and will exemplify what the OU Spanish team has done in an attempt to address such issues.

Foreign language teaching methodology has over the years changed according to the perceived needs of students at a particular moment in time. The approach towards the teaching of culture has also changed over time. Unfortunately, at a time when language methodology realised that students needed to become effective communicators and communicative approaches to language learning overtook previous methods, simulation and role playing left the language-teaching framework semi-empty of cultural content. As Fenner and Newby comment:

> *Over the past decades, however, textbooks have perhaps contained too little factual knowledge. Methodology has focused more on how to develop communicative skills from what might seem a bare minimum of cultural facts, and these facts have been mainly concerned with the everyday lives of*

150

representatives of the foreign language community, to a large extent the
everyday lives of young people. (Fenner and Newby, 2000: 145)

From the purely utilitarian point of view, in a global economy and, without going
very far, in a European market that wants to encourage mobility, language courses
suffer from a lack of cultural content that, if available would undoubtedly contribute
to students' better understanding of the cultures they may want to do business with,
and would certainly enhance their interpersonal communicative skills. Terry
Mughan notes that:

> *Current foreign language course design in higher education is questioned for its*
> *lack of focus on understanding people of other cultures. It is therefore argued*
> *that foreign language degree courses rapidly need to adopt an approach to*
> *intercultural learning which prepares students to move with more ease amongst*
> *numerous cultures and which is less bound, cognitively by the notion of the*
> *nation state.* (Mughan, 1999: 59)

2 What is 'culture' anyway?

According to the Hutchinson Encyclopaedia, culture is 'the way of life of a particular
society or group of people, including patterns of thought, beliefs, behaviour,
customs, traditions, rituals, dress and language, as well as art, music and literature'
(1994: 239). These are also the concepts likely to be conveyed by ordinary people
when asked what 'culture' means to them. Different disciplines, as well as different
perspectives or tendencies within them, approach the concept of culture from
different angles. For example, anthropologists are concerned with the concept of
culture as a shared heritage, while psychologists look at how an individual fits within
a set culture, be it their own or otherwise. In turn, a behaviourist would focus on the
shared and observable practices of a cultural group while a cognitivist would pay
attention to the shared ways of organising and interpreting the world. All the above
suggests that culture is not a simple concept and that each of its many aspects needs
to be taken into consideration to be able to learn about and interact successfully with
other cultures.

Language and culture are not separable. Language is no doubt the preferred code
used by human beings to communicate, and in this central role it becomes a crucial
component of cultural manifestations. Foreign-language teaching and learning are
concerned mainly with the development of communication among cultures.
Communication, however, goes beyond linguistic knowledge and is related to the
role that native and non-native participants play when interacting and their
perceptions of each other. Communication within a given culture is by nature a
complex process. In a given culture its members share a world where in general they

may share beliefs, meanings and sets of behaviours. However, the interaction amongst members requires that they continually negotiate a common understanding of events and such beliefs and behaviours, even though every culture 'imprints a value system upon the individual that grows up within it' (Brooks, 1964: 84). This value system makes it easier for members of a cultural group to perceive what gives them an important part of their cultural identity.

3 Communication across cultures

Just using the language competently doesn't mean being competent at interacting with the other culture:

> *When messages are transported across cultural boundaries they are encoded in one context and decoded in another.[…] This greatly increases the possibility of misunderstandings and of unexpected reactions.* (Smith 1966: 565)

This is why it is essential for students to develop skills that will enable them to achieve mutual cultural understanding, well beyond individual utterances.

In an attempt to describe the nature of this new educational dimension, various labels have already been proposed. They range from the concept of **sociolinguistic competence,** where the communicative teaching approach originated, and where equal emphasis is given to grammatical accuracy and appropriate use of language, to more recent labels such as **cross-cultural understanding, cultural awareness, sociocultural competence, intercultural competence** and **intercultural communicative competence.**

Each of these concepts considers the cultural dimension in a different light. Cross-cultural understanding means being able to feel empathy and easiness with people from another culture as well as being able to adapt one's own cultural heritage. The concept of cultural awareness highlights the importance of having a knowledge of the foreign culture, but also the need to have an analytical knowledge of one's own. Sociocultural competence, on the other hand, refers to a three-dimensional competence (pragmatic, cognitive and emotional) a language learner needs to develop so that he or she can interact effectively with the target culture. Van Ek's concept of communicative ability is the root of current perceptions of what it means to be an 'intercultural speaker' (Van Ek, 1986). It proposes that to be able to communicate effectively across cultures a speaker needs the right mix of linguistic, sociolinguistic, sociocultural and strategic competences. In other words, a holistic approach is required to become competent at communicating with other cultures.

Byram and Zarate's (1997) concept of interculturality has moved forward Van Ek's model. The idea has evolved into what Byram has identified as intercultural communicative competence (ICC) which comprises linguistic, sociolinguistic, discourse and a set of intercultural components. While Van Ek centres his ideal of communicative ability in the rules and parameters of the foreign culture and the native speaker, Byram (1997) considers that the culture of the foreign language learner plays an equally important role in the intercultural communicative process. Although in most contexts intercultural competence is synonymous with intercultural communicative competence, Byram makes a difference between the two. For him, the former refers to the interaction with another culture in the individual's own language, drawing on his or her knowledge of the foreign culture. The latter refers to the same type of interaction but in the language of the target culture.

But which language is used is not the only consideration implied when talking about interaction between cultures. Byram proposes that intercultural communicative competence (ICC) relates to the learner's ability to interact with people from other countries and cultures in the foreign language, as well as the ability to 'negotiate a mode of communication and interaction' or if necessary 'to act as mediator between people of different cultural origins and identities' (1997: 38). ICC prepares students to become effective communicators in a multicultural environment. The skills acquired by these communicators should be transferable to further situations across cultures. The multicultural speaker interacts beyond the situation or task in hand. He or she can maintain relationships with a multiplicity of other cultures beyond the communication exchange, and for this reason we will be referring to such competence as 'multicultural competence'.

4 A model for the development of multicultural competence

The ability to interact competently with another culture requires that in the context of foreign-language teaching there should be very specific cultural objectives. These objectives will vary according to the language in question, but as stated before, the skills acquired will be easily transferable from experiences with one culture or language to another. In the case of Spanish, the acquisition of a multicultural competence becomes a substantial objective since learners of the language are likely to interact not with a single culture, but with the vast spectrum of cultures which constitute the Spanish-speaking world today.

The above clearly suggests that several skills are needed to become multiculturally competent. The process involves the development of a range of sub-competences some linguistic, some social and some cultural. The success of intercultural interactions is based on the right combination of a number of factors: the effective exchange of information, the attitudes speakers will need to display to be able to compensate for any lack of knowledge of the other's culture or to allow for perceptions about facts and behaviour in the other culture to be different from his or her own. Cultural mismatches are unavoidable. The important thing is to be able to develop a positive attitude interested in different perspectives of cultural interpretation, a willingness to question one's own values and assumptions and to understand, interact with and even adapt to the other culture. This requires the development of skills that on the one hand allow for discovery and interpretation of evidence, events and facts, and on the other enable the foreign speaker to compare them with respective evidence, events and facts in his or her own environment. This experience will also extend knowledge and in turn will contribute to the development of the ability to interact, verbally and non-verbally, and to negotiate a role in the relationship that is being established with the interlocutor.

These concepts are developed in depth by Byram (1997) when he refers to the set of factors that play interdependent roles in the development of intercultural communicative competence. Such factors relate specifically to what multicultural speakers need to know about themselves and the foreign culture, the skills they need to analyse and relate to the foreign culture and their own, and the attitudes speakers need to develop so that successful multicultural interaction is assured.

Byram's model for ICC refers to the collection of competences involved:

- Attitudes (*savoir être*) relate to how a speaker approaches the other culture. Attitudes are normally referred to as positive or negative, but either way they can impact mutual understanding. Attitudes need to convey an open mind and a will to learn, discover and value the other culture;
- Knowledge (*savoir*) of the other culture and one's own and an understanding of what makes those cultures what they are: their history, their geographical or spatial boundaries, their institutions, the nature of social interactions, etc;
- Skills to be able to interpret and relate evidence, events and facts (*savoir comprendre*), to evaluate such data critically, allowing for perceptions different to one's own (*savoir s'engager*), to learn and discover (*savoir apprendre*) and finally, skills to engage successfully with the other culture (*savoir faire*).

5 From theory to practice

To be able to build a teaching model that develops the competences described above, the integration of a multicultural perspective in foreign-language programmes becomes an essential part of all the stages relevant to the teaching, learning and assessment process. It involves:

1. the formulation of cultural aims and outcomes during the curriculum-planning process;
2. the design of a syllabus showing quantifiable and achievable cultural objectives with corresponding assessment criteria;
3. the selection of varied authentic materials portraying crucial aspects of the foreign cultures;
4. the development of teaching methods that explicitly deal with and invite reflection upon cultural issues, as well as the development of learning strategies that enable learners to become multiculturally competent;
5. the evaluation of the achievement of cultural objectives.

An insight into the meaning of taking these steps can help us identify some important implications for teachers, learners and assessors. The inclusion of the multicultural dimension in the foreign languages curriculum means, in the first place, a change of focus from the traditionally dominant linguistic competence. This new focus sees language skills as an integral part of a wider educational context. The design of a cyclical curriculum in foreign languages where the same concepts, attitudes and skills are retaken at different stages seems to contribute effectively to the coherence of the learning process and to the continuous development of these cultural and sociolinguistic competences. This new context, however, requires accommodating new learning objectives in an already ambitious general language programme; it also entails furthering the educational responsibilities of the language teachers and assessors, ideally in liaison with other disciplines. All these adjustments are crucial and should not be overlooked.

The subsequent translation of the cultural elements into meaningful objectives in the foreign language syllabus and assessment criteria poses a number of challenges, such as the consideration of the learner's cultural profile (this being age, nationality, etc) and the presentation of the cultural variations within the communities who share the foreign language. The formulation of these objectives can be solved by moving away from restrictive ways of understanding language and culture, that is, from a description of a set of teacher and learner intentions. This model proposes the formulation of flexible objectives in terms of a range of skills, knowledge, attitudes, values and behaviour which may not always be observable and measurable.

The selection and use of authentic materials in foreign language learning is nowadays an established practice. However, as we have already pointed out, this practice does not necessarily imply the development of cultural competences. In fact, authentic texts (written and oral) and images continue to be culturally unexploited and are not being used as tools for the awakening of a multicultural awareness in language-learning environments. Two major questions arise: what to teach and how to develop teachers so that they are able to meet the requirements expected of them.

Culture, as we have already established, is a complicated concept. On the one hand, it manifests itself in different ways throughout the social strata, and on the other, it refers to constantly changing aspects of the various groups that constitute it. We cannot ignore the fact that a range of subcultures or variant cultural manifestations exists within a society, and that language plays a crucial role in the portrayal of these subcultures. Learning a foreign language needs to acknowledge and experience cultural diversity and ultimately contest traditional biases. For instance, exposure to different registers and accents in Spanish will help in understanding such linguistic varieties, in appreciating their contribution to what the Spanish language is today and as a result in presenting a balanced picture of the Hispanic cultures.

In addition, teaching requires an approach that doesn't present culture as a fixed body of knowledge but as a dynamic set of texts and images, each one opening a window into a combination of linguistic, social and cultural aspects of a particular group. Awareness of these facts is as crucial in learning about a culture as in teaching it. In this context, language teachers need to be culturally competent themselves and aware of their role in order to assist learners to develop the ability to engage effectively with other cultures. Teachers need to be willing to develop their own cultural competence, to be open-minded, to distance themselves from their own cultural world and to be willing to question their own prejudices and beliefs in order to succeed in carrying out their cultural responsibilities. Opportunities for teaching development in this area should be available.

Another important issue is that in a conventional language-learning situation, the acquisition of multicultural competence initially takes place in the classroom. Limiting the intercultural experience to this environment will to a great extent generate a decontextualised framework of action. For the context to be established, the experience therefore needs to go beyond the classroom, with teacher guidance, and from here to the 'real world' where students' autonomous skills will play a major role in the success of multicultural interaction. A gradual approach from the structured to the independent context, from the known to the unknown will make multicultural objectives realistically achievable.

6 Assessing multicultural competence

Assessment of the cultural competences still remains one of the greatest challenges. In the first place, items for assessment need to be identified in parallel with the definition of teaching objectives and we have already established the perceived difficulty in formulating such multicultural objectives. Secondly, although cultural knowledge and skills can be more easily measured, the assessment of progress in attitudes and values is even more difficult to carry out since attitudes on the whole are not quantifiable elements and usually involve personal ethical responses. However, this should not prevent language teachers from attempting other types of evaluation that in the long term may produce more positive results than those which can be quantified. One such method could be the creation of a varied portfolio or the integration of forms of self and peer-assessment that are formative rather than summative. Assessing multicultural progression may be easier in the context of a cyclical syllabus that encourages the development of knowledge, positive attitudes and interactive skills by revisiting topics or cultural aspects from a different angle at different levels.

Besides evaluating cultural competences, assessment also plays an essential role in their development. Assignments are in many cases the only elements of a course that are constantly renewed. They are, therefore, excellent means for the presentation of current cultural issues. The use of authentic materials in assignments can invite reflection upon changing aspects of a particular culture and the maintenance of a true picture of its dynamic nature.

7 The cultural dimension in the OU Spanish programme

The Spanish programme at the OU has applied the ICC model to develop a multicultural competence in adult learners who are studying at a distance. Firstly, the curriculum was conceived to include general and specific cultural objectives aiming at developing cultural versatility. The syllabus is thematic and raises cultural awareness through a balanced view of the Spanish-speaking communities around the world. It encourages the analysis of facts, events and data and the use of language which moves away from stereotypes. Samples of a wide range of authentic materials have been selected to facilitate a cultural encounter between the learner and the Hispanic communities. The exploitation of these authentic materials invites students to identify verbal and non-verbal signs in specific contexts. They encourage analysis, reflection and self-evaluation and emphasise the development of learner autonomy. The programme also includes a number of transferable academic skills intimately connected with cultural skills, such as the evaluation of the writer's attitude or the identification of facts, hypotheses and opinions. The expectation is that learners will acquire the ability to interact with the Spanish-speaking communities, to cope with possible cultural misunderstandings when they arise, to develop positive attitudes and to establish and maintain relationships with those who speak Spanish around the world.

The appendices which follow show samples of the kind of activities and assessment the OU Spanish programme has integrated to introduce the various factors that contribute to the development of a multicultural competence. The table in Appendix 1 presents a selection of topics covered in the OU Spanish courses and describes to what extent the activities around them focus on the development of the multicultural competence.

Appendix 2 shows a specific activity in the first-level Spanish course, *En rumbo*. In this instance the focus is on non-verbal communication. The purpose of this kind of cultural activity is not so much to encourage students to imitate natives' kinesics but to expose them to the role of non-verbal language in connection with the verbal discourse they are examining. The activity is based on a video sequence. First students are asked to pay attention to the meaning of what is said and then they are required to interpret a set of gestures and to reflect upon any possible similarities or differences with the gestures used in their own culture.

Appendix 3 presents a sample of assessment, a Tutor Marked Assignment (TMA), for the second-level Spanish course, *Viento en popa*. Here students are confronted with a real situation of conflict in a Latin-American country. This task requires them to play the role of a peacekeeper who has to write a report that establishes the need for dialogue between the two sides of the conflict and assesses the likelihood of success of the enterprise. From the reading of authentic documents produced by each side, students need to demonstrate in particular their interpretative skills and their ability to foresee the outcome based on the evidence, but also on their experience and own point of view.

8 Conclusion

The integration of a cultural dimension in the teaching and learning of a foreign language has important implications on all the stages of design and implementation of a language programme, and it concerns all the players in the teaching-learning process: course designers, authors, teachers, assessors, as well as institutions. Only a coherent approach will ensure that students are provided with optimum opportunities to become multiculturally competent speakers. Carrying out the process presents opportunities and challenges that, if addressed from the beginning of the development of a course, will not only guarantee the success of the enterprise but will also enrich the process and the final rewards for all concerned.

References

Brooks, N. (1964) *Language and language learning*. New York and Burlingame: Harcourt, Brace & World.

Byram, M. (1997) *Teaching and assessing intercultural communicative competence.* Clevedon: Multilingual Matters.

Byram, M. and Zarate, G. (1997) *The sociocultural and intercultural dimension of language learning and teaching.* Strasbourg: Council of Europe.

Byram, M., Zarate, G. and Neuner, G. (1998) *Sociocultural competence in language learning and teaching.* Strasbourg: Council of Europe.

Centre for Modern Languages, The Open University, *En rumbo.* (1999) London: Routledge.

Centre for Modern Languages, The Open University, (2000) *Viento en popa.* Milton Keynes: The Open University.

Education and Language Studies, The Open University, (2001) *A buen puerto.* Milton Keynes: The Open University.

Fenner, A. and Newby, D. (2000) *Approaches to materials design in European textbooks: implementing principles of authenticity, learner autonomy, cultural awareness.* European Centre for Modern Languages.

Hutchinson Encyclopaedia (1994) Netley, Australia: Helicon Publishing Ltd.

Mughan, T. (1999) 'Intercultural competence for foreign language students in higher education' in *Language learning journal, 20*: 59–65.

Nemetz-Robinson, G. L. (1985) *Cross-cultural understanding.* New York: Pergamon Institute of English.

Parry, M. (1998) 'The Renaissance dream: literary and anthropological perspectives on cross-cultural capability' in Killick, D. and Parry, M. (eds) *Cross-cultural capability: the why, the ways and the means: new theories and methodologies in language education.* Leeds: Leeds Metropolitan University.

Smith, A. (1966) *Communication and culture.* New York: Holt, Rinehart and Winston.

Trim, J. L. M. (1993) Document CC-LANG (93) 2. Strasbourg: Council of Europe.

Van Ek, J. (1986) *Objectives for foreign language learning.* Strasbourg: Council of Europe.

Van Ek, J. and Trim, J. L. M. (1991) *Threshold level 1990.* Strasbourg: Council of Europe.

Appendix 1

Sample of activities from the Spanish programme and their multicultural exploitation

TOPIC	KNOWLEDGE	ATTITUDES	SKILLS
Introduction to the concept of multiculturalism	The origins and identity of the various Spanish-speaking cultures	Curiosity; interest in finding out the make-up of the various Spanish-speaking communities	Discovering and identifying significant references that highlight the main milestones in the history of the Spanish-speaking people
The Cuban revolution	Cuban history and the make up of today's Cuba	Openness; interest in finding out the development of Cuba as a nation and a cultural entity; questioning own perceptions and beliefs	Interpreting, relating and identifying references that explain the nature of the relationship between Cuba and the rest of the world
Tú or *Usted*	Grammatical knowledge; concept of register; modes of address	Willingness to engage with Spanish speakers, negotiate a role in the interaction and if necessary be a mediator in the intercultural communicative process	Discovering rules of behaviour and interaction, relating to own culture and engaging with Spanish speakers, negotiating a suitable role in the communicative process according to the circumstances
Speaking with your hands	Non-verbal communication; Conventions and register	Readiness to engage in verbal and non-verbal exchanges	Discovering, relating, interpreting and interacting appropriately with Spanish speakers
Task for assessment	Colombian history; factual information about Colombia today	Interest in discovering perspectives of interpretation of familiar and unfamiliar phenomena which may be different from the student's own; questioning own perceptions and beliefs	Identifying ethnocentric perspectives in a document; interpreting information and relating it to own cultural experience

Appendix 2

Activity from *En Rumbo 4*, Unit 1, Session 3

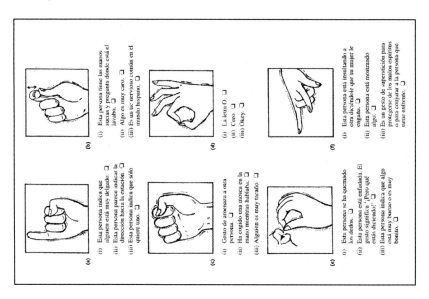

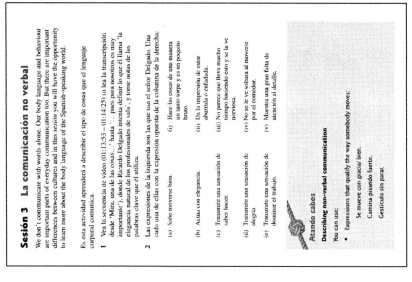

Sesión 3   La comunicación no verbal

We don't communicate with words alone. Our body language and behaviour are important parts of everyday communication too. But there are important differences between cultures and in this *sesión* you will have the opportunity to learn more about the body language of the Spanish-speaking world.

En esta actividad aprenderá a describir el tipo de cosas que el lenguaje corporal comunica.

1 Vea la secuencia de vídeo (01:13:53 – 01:14:25) (o lea la transcripción desde 'Mira, una de las cosas...' hasta '...pues para nosotros es muy importante'), donde Ricardo Delgado intenta definir lo que él llama 'la elegancia natural de los profesionales de sala', y tome notas de las palabras clave que él utiliza.

2 Las expresiones de la izquierda son las que usa el señor Delgado. Una cada una de ellas con la expresión opuesta de la columna de la derecha:

(a) Sabe moverse bien.

(b) Actúa con elegancia.

(c) Transmite una sensación de saber hacer.

(d) Transmite una sensación de alegría.

(e) Transmite una sensación de dominar el trabajo.

(i) Hace las cosas de una manera un tanto torpe y es un poquito bruto.

(ii) Da la impresión de estar aburrida o enfadada.

(iii) No parece que lleve mucho tiempo haciendo esto y se la ve nerviosa.

(iv) No se le ve con soltura al moverse por el comedor.

(v) Muestra una gran falta de atención al detalle.

Atando cabos

Describing non-verbal communication

You can use:

• Expressions that qualify the way somebody moves:

Se mueve con gracia/ bien.

Camina pisando fuerte.

Gesticula sin parar.

© The Open University 1995

Appendix 3

Extract from Tutor Marked Assignment (TMA 09), *Viento en popa*, 2000 (© The Open Unviversity)

EVALUACIÓN ESCRITA

En esta evaluación va a escribir un informe dirigido a la dirección de la organización internacional para la que trabaja. La labor de esta organización es la promoción de iniciativas de paz en el Tercer Mundo.

El informe debe argumentar la necesidad de establecer un diálogo entre el Gobierno colombiano y las Fuerzas Armadas Revolucionarias de Colombia (FARC), para poner fin a la lucha armada que ha padecido este país durante más de cinco décadas. Su informe deberá basarse en los dos textos que siguen (Texto A y Texto B).

1. Lea los dos textos. El Texto A representa los puntos de vista del Gobierno colombiano. El Texto B representa el punto de vista de las Fuerzas Armadas Revolucionarias de Colombia.
2. Redacte un informe en español de entre 400 y 500 palabras. El informe deberá tener un registro formal y deberá incluir los siguientes puntos:
   * Información sobre el origen del conflicto;
   * los objetivos que las dos partes tienen en común;
   * los cambios que deben ocurrir según cada una de las partes del conflicto;
   * su opinión personal sobre la importancia del diálogo para alcanzar la paz;
   * una valoración personal, justificada sobre las posibilidades que hay de que estos grupos lleguen a un acuerdo.

TEXTO A

Testimonio del Presidente de la República

Colombianos, hoy venimos a cumplir una cita con la historia. Hemos demorado casi medio siglo en hacerla realidad. Sabemos que los ojos de todos, de cada trabajador, de cada empresario, de cada campesino, de cada madre de familia, de cada soldado, de cada desplazado, de cada insurgente están pendientes de nosotros.

Los colombianos somos conscientes de que un conflicto de muchas décadas no se va a terminar en unos pocos meses, pero yo estoy seguro de que al culminar la ruta que nos hemos trazado lograremos la reconciliación nacional. Como presidente de todos los colombianos quiero una nación próspera y optimista, sin violencia, comprometida contra la corrupción, progresando contra la pobreza y con sus mejores esfuerzos dedicados al bienestar de mis compatriotas. En esta tarea de cambio se encuentra empeñado mi gobierno. Luchamos de manera infatigable contra la pobreza y contra la corrupción, buscamos crear las condiciones para dar empleo seguro y confiable, diseñamos un plan de desarrollo para construir la paz y fortalecer la imagen de Colombia en el exterior.

Retomemos las palas y los azadones, los libros y cuadernos, los martillos y los ladrillos para construir el país que todos queremos.

Hay quienes no han visto que la 'guerra de la paz' se gana en el empleo, en la vivienda, en la nutrición, en la salud, en el respeto a la ecología, en el respeto a la vida.

TEXTO B

Testimonio de las Fuerzas Armadas Revolucionarias de Colombia (FARC)

En 1964, a raíz de la Revolución Cubana, el presidente Kennedy diseñó un plan contrainsurgente para América Latina, con el fin de evitar el surgimiento de otras revoluciones en el Continente; a estas medidas diseñadas por el Pentágono se les dio el nombre de Plan Lasso, y fue dentro de este marco que se les declaró la guerra a 48 campesinos colombianos. En aquel entonces esos 48 campesinos solamente exigían la construcción de vías de penetración para sacar sus productos agrícolas, un centro de mercadeo, unas escuelas para educar a sus hijos, un centro de asistencia sanitaria y libertad de movilizarse sin estar siempre atemorizados por los abusos de la policía y el ejército.

Ante la inminencia de la agresión gubernamental, estos 48 hombres se dirigieron, sin ningún éxito, al propio presidente, al Congreso, a los gobernadores, a la Cruz Roja nacional e internacional, a la Iglesia, a las Naciones Unidas, a los intelectuales franceses y demás organizaciones democráticas, para que impidieran el comienzo de una nueva confrontación armada en Colombia con imprevisibles consecuencias.

Consideramos que, para ambientar el proceso de paz que hoy se inicia, es necesario que nuestros adversarios terminen con el lenguaje calumnioso de bandidos, terroristas, narcotraficantes, bandoleros, etc., porque la confrontación no se gana con insultos, sino haciendo una sociedad más justa y terminando con las causas objetivas de la violencia.

Queremos paz sin hambre, sin leyes represivas, sin mordaza a la prensa, con tierra, salud, vivienda, bienestar, empleo, crecimiento.

Glossary

AFLS	Association for French Language Studies
ALLADIN	Autonomous Language Learning in Art and Design using Interactive Networks (TLTP Project)
ALMS	Autonomous Learning Modules, Helsinki University
CALL	Computer-Aided Language Learning
CEQ	Course Evaluation Questionnaire
CERCLES	*Confédération Européenne des Centres de Langues de l'Enseignement Supérieur*
CHED	Centre for Higher Education Development, Coventry University
CIEL	Curriculum and Independence for the Learner Support Network (FDTL Project)
CILT	Centre for Information on Language Teaching and Research
CLCS	Centre for Language and Communication Studies, Trinity College Dublin
DEVELOP	Developing Excellence in Language Teaching through the Observation of Peers (FDTL Project)
DHFETE	Department of Higher and Further Education, Training and Employment (Northern Ireland)
DOPLA	Development of Postgraduate and Language Assistants (FDTL Project)
EFL	English as a Foreign Language
ELC	European Language Council
ELP	European Language Portfolio
ESL	English as a Second Language
FDTL	Fund for the Development of Teaching and Learning
FDTL-CGL	FDTL Co-ordinating Group for Languages
HE	Higher Education
HEFCE	Higher Education Funding Council for England
HEFCW	Higher Education Funding Council for Wales
HEQC	Higher Education Quality Council
HESA	Higher Education Statistical Agency
ICC	Intercultural Communicative Competence
ILT	Institute for Learning and Teaching in Higher Education
IWLP	Institution-Wide Languages Programme

L1	First Language
L2	Second Language
LARA	Learning and Residence Abroad (FDTL Project)
LTSN	Learning and Teaching Support Network
MLTC	Modern Languages Teaching Centre, University of Sheffield
MOO	Multi-user domain, Object Oriented (virtual environment)
NCT	National Co-ordination Team for the Teaching Quality Enhancement Fund
QA	Quality Assessment
QAA	Quality Assurance Agency for Higher Education
RAPPORT	Residence Abroad Project at Portsmouth (FDTL Project)
SCHML	Standing Conference of Heads of Modern Languages in Universities
SHEFC	Scottish Higher Education Funding Council
SMILE	Strategies for Managing the Independent Learning Environment (FDTL Project)
TL	Target Language
TLTP	Teaching and Learning Technology Programme
TQA	Teaching Quality Assessment (informal nickname for Quality Assessment process)
TQEF	Teaching Quality Enhancement Fund
TransLang	Transferable Skills Development for Non-specialist Learners of Modern Languages (FDTL Project)
UCAS	Universities and Colleges Admissions Service
UCML	University Council of Modern Languages
WELL	Web-Enhanced Language Learning (FDTL Project)

Contributors

Inma Álvarez is a lecturer in Spanish at the Open University. She also has taught Spanish in the United States and other UK universities. Her research interests are in the field of the development of cultural awareness in language programmes. She has worked on the integration of such awareness into the Open University's third-level Spanish course, *A buen puerto* and is currently researching the role of translation skills in the development of intercultural skills.

Mark Bannister is Professor of French at Oxford Brookes University and has published widely on the evolution of ethical and ideological *mentalités* in France throughout the seventeenth century. Since 1997 he has also been Director of the Learning and Residence Abroad (LARA) Project, funded by HEFCE.

Jim Coleman is a specialist in university language teaching and learning, with a dozen authored or edited books and eighty articles to his name. He has also written French course materials and books on early French literature. From 1997–2001 he co-ordinated the government-funded Residence Abroad Project. After nine years as Professor at the University of Portsmouth, he moves in 2001 to a new Chair of Language Learning and Teaching at the Open University.

Glynis Cousin is a Senior Research Fellow in the Centre for Higher Education Development (CHED), Coventry University. She supports the building of pedagogic research capacity across disciplines at Coventry and as Research Associate on a nationally-funded programme which is exploring the enhancement of teaching and learning in undergraduate education (with Edinburgh, Durham and Napier Universities).

Vicky Davies is currently the Open Learning Adviser for Languages at the University of Ulster and is shortly to take up the post of Teaching Development Adviser at the same institution. She is the author of a number of vocationally-oriented language textbooks and her current research interests are autonomous learning, reflection in teaching and learning and transferable skills.

Derrik Ferney is Associate Dean of the School of Languages and Social Sciences at Anglia Polytechnic University. His main interests are computer-assisted language learning and institution-Wide Languages Programmes. He has recently co-edited *Current trends in modern languages for non-specialist linguists* (CILT, 2000), and co-authored Langenscheidt's *Wortschatz Wirtschaftsenglisch* (2000) and accompanying *Business Englisch Wortschatztraining* (2001).

Cecilia Garrido is the Head of Spanish at the Open University. She has extensive teaching experience both in South America and the UK. She has been responsible for the development of the Spanish programme at the OU, with a focus on the teaching of Spanish as a world language. Her main research interests are related to the development of intercultural competence and the implications for teachers, students and course designers.

David Head is Professor of International Business Communication and Head of the Department of International Business in the Plymouth Business School, University of Plymouth. He is the author of *'Made in Germany': the corporate identity of a nation* (1992) and co-author of the *Harrap German Business Management Dictionary* (1999).

Sarah Hudspith is Lecturer in Russian at The University of Leeds. In September 2000 she successfully defended her PhD on the subject of 'Dostoevsky and Slavophilism: A new perspective on unity and brotherhood'. A specialist in nineteenth-century Russian literature, she is also interested in foreign language learning and CALL.

Michael Jones is Director of the Languages Resource Unit at the University of Ulster, and Senior Lecturer in German. His research interests are currently divided between ICT in language learning, *ab initio* teaching and the German resistance to Hitler.

David Little is Director of the Centre for Language and Communication Studies and Associate Professor of Applied Linguistics at Trinity College, Dublin. His principal research interest is the theory and practical implementation of learner autonomy in the second/foreign language classroom, on which he has published widely.

Nicole McBride is Principal Lecturer in French at the University of North London. Her main research interests are in the area of language learning and teaching. She has published French course materials and books as well as articles on CALL, grammar and hypertext and is currently developing on-line teaching materials. She recently co-edited a book investigating the relationship of language and culture in language degrees, *Target culture – target language?*.

John Morley teaches on the in-sessional EAP programmes at the University of Manchester and co-co-ordinates the credit-rated tandem programme there. He has an MEd (Hons) from the University of New England and has previously worked in Australia, Singapore, Spain and Indonesia. His main interests are learner autonomy and genre text analysis of written texts.

Marina Orsini-Jones is Subject Leader for Italian in the School of International Studies and Law at Coventry University. She has been involved in focus group research about motivation in language learning since 1997. She is furthermore carrying out research on the integration of the virtual learning environment WebCT in the languages curriculum. She has published various articles about collaborative learning environments for language learning and a CD-ROM to teach Italian language, culture and society. She has also published in the field of contemporary Italian studies, with particular reference to immigrant women in Italy.

Rob Rix is Head of Modern Languages at Trinity and All Saints College, Leeds. He has worked principally on professional task-based teaching, learning and assessment techniques, listening skills and hypermedia applications in language learning.

Nicola Reimann is Senior Lecturer in German at the University of Sunderland and is currently teaching German as a Foreign Language at the *Freie Universität Berlin* in Germany. She has specialised in foreign language pedagogy and language classroom research and has recently completed a PhD on 'Non-continuation on an Institution-Wide Languages Programme'. She is interested in non-specialist and beginners' language provision in HE and has co-edited and contributed to a volume devoted to *ab initio* language learning and teaching.

Sandra Truscott is Senior Lecturer in Languages at the University of Manchester and Director of the Languagewise programme. She has an MA and PhD in Latin-American Literature from the University of London. She is Director of the Languagewise programme and Programme Head in Modern Languages for the Centre of Continuing Education. Her main interests are contemporary Spain and educational methodology.

Lesley Walker is French co-ordinator at the Modern Languages Teaching Centre, University of Sheffield. She is a trained teacher and assessor. She has research interests in the use of the new technologies in language learning and teaching, and the role of learner strategies in second-language acquisition. She has published on various aspects of learner autonomy and tandem learning.